PHYSIQUE AFTER 50

Scott Abel

Edited by Perry Mykleby

Published in by:

Scott Abel

© Copyright 2016

ISBN-13: **978-1539497738**
ISBN-10: **1539497739**

Disclaimer

Please consult your family physician or healthcare provider before beginning any new exercise or training program.

The information provided in this book is intended as a resource, and is not to be used or relied upon as medical advice, or as a substitute for medical advice. The information provided in this book is to be used at the sole discretion and risk of the reader.

Table of Contents

Introduction

A former client of mine is just turned 60. He writes me now in desperation, trying to continue the hardcore bodybuilding lifestyle we shared back when we were in our mid 30s.

This guy stayed on steroids long after many others would have, because he wanted to keep competing — right into his late 50s.

But all didn't go well for him with this hardcore, never-give-it-up approach. He has had two shoulder surgeries. He has torn both triceps. One biceps had to be reattached surgically. He has had one knee and both hips replaced.

In short, his body is very, very broken. And, as is so often the case for an online coach, it's only NOW he writes me for help!

He was under the misguided idea that taking testosterone and growth hormone would keep him young. However, they ended up contributing to the wear and tear of his body.

Contrary to what many might think, it wasn't only drugs. A lot of it has to do with something much simpler and something far, far more common. He was trying to maintain same kind of training regimen we both used when we were younger, long after he should have seriously adjusted his program to protect his body, his joints, his hormones and more.

Ultimately, that was his biggest mistake.

* * *

Another former client writes me. He once competed at a very lean, ripped 185 lbs. and now weighs almost 400 lbs.

He has many of the health problems, like diabetes, often associated with that kind of obesity. At 53 years old, he is too heavy to properly exercise (especially the kind of exercise he was used to).

He can't even work, so his wife must support the family financially. He is effectively disabled because of his weight and his health problems. And she is exhausted from working and taking care of him as well.

Fewer than 20 years ago, he competed in bodybuilding contests. He was showing off his physique, aspiring to the classical proportions of Greek statues of the gods and the Olympians.

These days he takes morphine for diabetic nerve pain. The morphine leaves him drowsy and out of it. He worries he may be abusing it. In total, he takes between 12 and 15 medications daily, some of which are simply to counteract the side effects of the others.

And it's only *now* is when he writes me for help!

Both of these former clients feel like they are in a life and death situation.

* * *

Let's juxtapose these two former clients with two gentlemen from my local gym.

These two guys were kind enough to join me in recording a few videos to support a "Welcome to the Platinum Club" article I wrote on my blog.

These two men, Mike and Rick, are 62 and 60 respectively. They work out very diligently, and by "diligently," I mean intelligently and routinely.

Mike, 62, is a long-distance cyclist. We both live in Kelowna, British Columbia, near the west coast of Canada. It's hilly and mountainous here. Being a long-distance cyclist says a lot.

Rick, 60, is a land developer and he is working (happily) as productively as ever.

Mike brags about keeping up with his grandkids. Rick talks about the way his son invites him along with his friends for weekend activity trips.

Both Mike and Rick have killer physiques. They *look* healthy. These two guys exemplify what I call membership in The Platinum Club.

I have now contrasted four different people over the age of 50. These examples were meant to illustrate some of the differences you can experience, depending upon how you take care of your body as you age.

* * *

Let's talk about what happens to your body as you approach your fifth decade of life.

No one – *no one* – is exempt from the passage of years.

Every year after the age of 25, the average North American gains about one pound of total body weight, while losing one-third to one-half pound of muscle. This is why even professional athletes are done with their careers, or see their performance on the decline, as early as their mid-30s in some sports. Without some form of resistance training to offset this reality, most people experience at least a 30% loss of muscle before the age 70. Compounding the muscle loss, people tend to become less active: less muscle combined with more bodyweight makes activity more difficult and more exhausting.

Women, unfortunately, are at an even greater disadvantage. The most recent research shows that women on average lose muscle *twice* as fast as men the same age. This can of course make a huge difference in their ability to maintain an ideal, or much less, a preferred body weight.

Furthermore, the loss of estrogen after menopause can create even more challenges to women's metabolism, handicapping their body's innate ability to regulate overall bodyweight and appetite, or use energy for lean tissue building rather than store it as fat.

* * *

The population as a whole is aging. And yet there aren't many experts in the fitness industry speaking directly to the over-50 crowd.

Most fitness "knowledge" takes a one-size-fits-all approach. That approach just doesn't apply to you at all, with all that is happening in your body as you pass the age of 50.

Let's face it: most of "fitness and diet" is a younger person's game. That is an industry bias, dictated by profit and loss, and by teams of marketers. This moneymaking focus leads to all sorts of other biases and blind spots, but what's relevant here is that they are not speaking to you, the over-50 crowd. (Ironically, as the over-50 market grows, it becomes more and more commercially viable. Regardless, the industry maintains its youth bias.)

* * *

I'll admit there was a time when I was guilty of this myself. I didn't appreciate the changes that go on in the body until I experienced it *for* myself. The changes that go on in your body as you approach and pass that 50-year mark are unique and very different than the changes you experience as you transition from your 20s to your 30s, and then into your 40s.

When I first pitched the idea for this book, my business advisor suggested I call it "Physique After 40," to speak to a wider demographic. I did consider it, but only for about 10 minutes. I wrote him an email back, saying "no way." If you are over 50 and reading this, then you might know why I couldn't do that.

I was still guest posing at age 44. Well into my 40s my body fat was about 10%, yet I still weighed over 250 lbs. But as my 40s wore on, and as I transitioned into my 50s, there was no way I could maintain that size or that physique in a healthy way. (You can perhaps squeeze in a *few* extra years by doing it in an unhealthy way, but I assure you: there *will* be consequences.)

As I approached 50, things changed: my body started breaking down. I had to adjust my training, and some aspects of my lifestyle, to account for this.

I could live with not guest posing any longer, and I could therefore live with not maintaining huge amounts of muscle at a relatively low body fat.

But let's also be real: I still wanted to look good and *feel* good. My training is very important to me. I didn't want to let that go, nor did I want to let go of any of the benefits that intelligent training provides.

* * *

The Platinum Club

The Platinum Club is a group whose only requirements are being over the age of 50, and being in wise pursuit of physical fitness and excellent physique. Why Platinum? Platinum is more valuable than both silver and gold.

No application fees are necessary, other than the work you'll need to do to qualify and stay a member. And believe me, membership has its privileges: looking better—maybe even younger, feeling better physically and mentally, better sex life, less chance of age or obesity discrimination in the workplace.

The idea behind the Platinum Club is to get past settling for the "Golden Years." This idea first started percolating in my mind a few years ago. The many realities of my own body changing, and appeals for help from former clients, prompted me. Plus, no fitness author seems to be paying any attention to this unique demographic, as witnessed by the one-size-fits-all approach to training you can see everywhere.

It's possible to work out for a better physique –

and a better-*looking* physique – after 50 if you do it right. You just have to go about it correctly, and accept things about your body that other people won't understand if they are not themselves over 50 years of age "Physique after 50" is not just simply a cosmetic solution for our age group. It's also a cautionary tale of what happens when people let life get ahead of them. They end up leading "reactive" lives, rather than lives of design. It's a cautionary tale that you will hear me repeat often as I address The Platinum Club:

"Make time for wellness, or make time for illness."

I begin here with 'Physique After 50' because of what I witness when I help people focus on looking better. When they begin to look better, they get inspired, which then motivates them to continue. Physique After 50 and Platinum Club membership is about *changing your mind* about your age.

You may be reading this having eased through life with no diet routine, no workout regimen, or no fitness lifestyle previously. You've now realized that you are paying dearly for it now that you're over 50. Lifestyle habits are very, VERY hard things to break, or re-create. Eating whatever you want, and not treating your body well nutritionally, combined with adequate sleep hygiene, comes back to haunt you a lot more intensely once you are in your 50s. You may even be surprised by medical problems that have occurred suddenly, or gradually, as a result. Physique After 50 is about health first and foremost.

I've recently had several occasions to gather with people my age who I've known for a while. Some have held up well; others have not. The ones who have not held up well looked much older than they actually are. But you can also tell they feel much older than they are by the way they carry themselves. What stuck out to me were the topics of conversations among those who aged well versus those who did not. The ones who did not age well seemed to talk about specific ailments.

There are millions of people around the globe who have lived long lives without ever working out, or exercising in any real way. Research about exercise's contribution to longevity is cloudy at best. The conversation should include adding life to your years. I witnessed in my own parents the effects of an unhealthy lifestyle, of poor diet and lack of exercise, and the eventual impediment that that kind of lifestyle puts in someone's quality of life as they age.

As my father was dying of congestive heart failure, the result of more than 70 years of smoking, a poor diet, and no exercise regimen to speak of, my friend and colleague Kevin Weiss showed me a picture of a man my father's age competing in a powerlifting event. That is the kind of juxtaposition you should consider here. The fitness lifestyle isn't about living longer; it's about living better with the time you are given.

It's never too late to treat your body better.

The fitness lifestyle has the power to change your life, but it requires investment in your body. If you can't be bothered because it all seems like too much work, then ask yourself if staying on your current path is giving you the life and body you want.

You don't just have to sit back and invite accelerated and pre-mature aging. You can choose to dive directly into a better life for yourself. You can choose to join The Platinum Club, where membership has its privileges. Physique After 50 examines how to optimize the body you have now.

You shouldn't expect too little of the aging body and physique; nor should you expect far too much out of them. So, in Physique After 50, we will cover:

- How to sculpt a better physique, even after 50
- How you can get invigorated by exercise and achieve health and appearance benefits
- Methods to work around your limitations, ease joint and muscle pain, guard against Type 2 diabetes and heart disease

- That not every exercise is good exercise
- Intelligent, strategic, traditional body part bodybuilding type training protocol (innervation training) will help you achieve these goals.

Looking better, and feeling better– *that* is the promise of this book!

Being over 50 doesn't have to mean it's time for you to just "settle" for your golden years. It is absolutely still possible to add some sculpted muscle to your physique, if you are smart and realistic with your exercise protocol. And the smarter and more intelligent you are with your exercise protocol, the more you will reap the benefits of this smarter more intelligent approach as you age. This book will show you how.

Chapter 1.

The Realities of Aging, Muscle Loss and Sarcopenia

Like many of you reading this, I "joined" The Platinum Club begrudgingly. I had no idea how much my own inner physiology would change between the ages of 40 and 50. But change it did, and drastically. And like many of you, those nagging injuries—big or small—from earlier years turned into painful limitations for me as the years passed.

In 2000, when I was 39, I required back surgery to remove two discs from my lumbar spine. For a few years afterwards, I had dependency issues with painkillers. But now, I am hard pressed to be convinced to even take an aspirin for a headache. I completely recovered over the course of two years, but now at age 55, this area of my back is something I have to guard. (I even wear a supportive back brace for my power walks. Although I can work out vigorously with weights with no problem, my back simply doesn't like the "jarring motion" of even walking fast.)

Then, in my early 40s, I began experiencing shoulder point pain and limited range of motion and function. By my late 40s, I had to rearrange my cupboards in my kitchen because I couldn't confidently reach above my head for glasses and bowls, etc. I ended up getting the maximum cortisone shot dosage allowed, and yet only that first cortisone shot gave me any true relief.

I was scheduled for shoulder replacement surgery, which would likely have ended my workout routines, at least as I had known them. The surgeon told me that the shoulder joint isn't meant to lift anything too heavy overhead. When I shared with the surgeon that I had used shoulder presses with 110 lb. dumbbells, he responded that I was now paying the price.

I am no orthopedist by any means, but I am a smart guy and an expert in exercise and training science. I knew that maintaining my fitness lifestyle required my brain and expertise to re-craft things. So I developed this working statement:

Train your age, not your experience.

Aging is a fact that must be considered in your exercise regimen as you approach age 50 and beyond. It took a couple years of experimenting, but I came up with some very sound methodologies for training after age 50 that use traditional body part innervation protocols. My popular Hard Gainer Solution program, and my own current 6 Day PA50 training protocol, are examples. I also discovered the value of proper warm-ups for the joints—and the value of rotator cuff work for me specifically—in order to rehab and "prehab" my damaged shoulders.

So, even at our age, it is common knowledge that weight training prevents injuries, prevents or helps control arthritis, prevents loss of bone density, and fights off a host of other issues that often happen as people age.

For women in particular, the more lean tissue you add the healthier you will be and the better you will look and the more robust your metabolism will be. The mistake most women over 50 continue to make is focusing on losing body fat by engaging in calorie-consuming activities. But these kinds of activities break down muscle, not build it up, adding to the consequences of the aging process already underway. That mentality of "calorie-burning first" only invites accelerated and premature aging. Like men, women would be far better off to use resistance training with the goal of physique-sculpting, and replace the mistaken notion of calorie-burning and fat loss.

Coincidentally enough, I just finished watching a documentary called "The Resurrection of Jake Roberts." It is about former professional wrestlers Jake Roberts and Scott Hall, attempting to overcome drug and alcohol abuse, and deal with tremendous pain and physical limitations brought on in their younger years and exacerbated as they aged. It was sad to see the effect of a broken down body on the mind and emotional wellness. It was yet another cautionary tale of what can happen if you take your body for granted in your younger years.

A word about meds

Chronic injuries and limitations affect the hormonal and biochemical environments at our age. Injuries or chronic conditions brought about by decades of training always involve inflammation. Some inflammation is unavoidable in the aging process. Too much is never good, so medications may indeed be required. I take Celebrex for my arthritis, but not because I'm hoping it will cure pain and inflammation. I took it upon myself to use my expertise to find other cures and methods. And while I still take Celebrex, I can easily reach over my head pain-free now, and my shoulders are no longer a big limitation. This is how an intelligently designed, "proper," training protocol can combat and relieve some of the more dismal effects of aging.

Like I did with my osteoarthritis, you can 'treat' pain and inflammation and manage it medically, while weight training the right way to reduce pain and inflammation – to make your muscles stronger surrounding the joint, which then support the joint better.

I'm not an advocate for natural remedies. It was when I *stopped* taking fish oils that my shoulder pain was reduced. I don't understand the "tree-hugger" mentality in the fitness industry that is suspicious of medical intervention, yet promotes useless supplements and alternative therapies.

Muscle Loss and "Sarcopenia"

If you are over 50 it's important that you know what "sarcopenia" means. Sarcopenia is all about the loss of muscle mass as we age.

Serious muscular growth for anyone 50 years old and above is doubtful. And you shouldn't want to add lots of extra muscle mass at this age anyway – to do so is a systemic stress just as hard on the body as gaining extra body fat weight would be. For me, dropping some 30 to 40 lbs. of muscle freed my joints from pain and pressure. So while it's not smart to try to add say, 20 lbs. of muscle to your physique after age 50, you can certainly aim instead for "mass with class," and for a sculpted, balanced, and aesthetically-pleasing physique. This is completely possible for both men and women over 50.

To make matters worse, the loss of muscle mass, that increases as we age, negatively impacts metabolism. Diminishing muscle mass and muscle density contributes to metabolic slowdown, especially if you have never really done resistance training before. Metabolism slows down on its own even separate from all the other aging processes that contribute to it. And it should also be no surprise to you that there is slower recovery from exercise in general as you age, accompanied by more everyday achy-ness, even from more mundane activities if your body is unaccustomed to them.

As you can guess, loss of muscle mass also means declining strength as we age. For this reason, you shouldn't be comparing your abilities and physical self to your younger years. Those years are gone and you have a new reality to face. The good news here is that for those of you who have previously not done much working out with weights, if you do the right kind of resistance training exercise, you will experience an even more pronounced positive effect – positive for muscle function, and positive for metabolism.

Educating people on these realities is difficult. If you do a general Google search for "how much does metabolism slow down with age," you end up with a lot of fitness industry biased nonsense about "prevention" and the like. Articles like these are very misleading.

Sarcopenia presents a host of issues that include weakness, fatigue, lack of stamina, lack of vitality and verve, diabetes, and effects of previous injuries. There are several that deserve focus.

Limited ROM

Sarcopenia leads to ROM (range of motion) limitations in certain areas of the body in general or for specific exercises. This is due in large part to gradual joint enlargement, obstruction from bony changes, diminished joint flexibility, and reduced ligament tenacity. These are separate from the overall loss of muscle that happens as you age, and speeds up decade after decade after your 40s. All of these factors must be considered into realistic exercise performance after age 50.

Cosmetic

There are cosmetic effects to consider here as well. The tight skin tone of your youth gives way to looseness, and your skin becomes less elastic and you accumulate wrinkles. I often joke that parts of my skin look like a Shar-Pei dog now when I pull my skin out near my elbows for instance, I have all this loose wrinkly skin that doesn't just snap back like it used to. This is normal.

Hormonal

After age 50 is when you really tend to feel the consequences of the natural, age-related decreases of certain hormones. Growth hormone decreases affect both genders. Testosterone decreases affect men more so than women. IGF, Insulin-like-Growth-Factor also decreases as well, which can have an effect on your susceptibility to diabetes. All these hormones decrease as you age, and the combined effect means more metabolic slowdown, and more difficulty controlling body fat and regulating your bodyweight.

Obviously, women in their 50s are now into menopause and many of them experience dire effects of that, while some only experience very mild changes. The decade of your 50s is when you will notice the greatest changes beginning to happen to your body as a result of aging.

Reduction in nerve cells

One of the lesser-known effects of sarcopenia is age-related reduction in nerve cells responsible for sending signals from the brain to the muscles to initiate movement. This can make it harder to learn exercises and make it harder for your body to adapt to various forms of new exercise. This is one reason why it is not a good idea to force high intensity training on people over 50 who are just learning to use weights.

Diminished protein synthesis

Because of age-related metabolic and biochemical changes, there is also a decrease in the body's ability to synthesize protein. This is also most noticeable from age 50 onward. And if you don't control this as you age into your 60s and 70s, you will experience an inadequate ability to take in enough calories and/or protein to sustain muscle mass. We all know older adults who are told to drink Ensure and other concoctions to try to offset these more pernicious effects of the aging process.

You should be familiar with all these effects of sarcopenia. How you deal with them is the difference between Platinum Club membership and experiencing their more debilitating effects. A little prevention work with diet and exercise goes a long, long way in terms of quality of life after 50.

Treatments for Sarcopenia

Experts almost unanimously agree that exercise is the main treatment for combating the effects of sarcopenia. But this is far too general in scope. Experts who go into greater depth on the subject make sure to clarify that the type of exercise that is best for combating sarcopenia is **resistance training**. That said, many of these experts equate resistance training with strength training. Resistance training and strength training are not the same. Pure strength training of the powerlifting type is done for low reps and heavy loads, and usually with barbells. Many trainees over 50 will experience way too much pain and injury risk from trying to lift this way. In my expert opinion, strength-density training, using the traditional bodybuilding approach, makes the most sense if you are over 50.

Resistance training has positive effects on the neuromuscular system, the biochemical system, hormonal concentrations and even positive protein synthesis rates. This latter effect is especially important for optimizing metabolism as you age.

Most experts *do not* recommend doing a lot of aerobic/cardio work to fight off sarcopenia. If your goal is a robust and healthy "physique after 50," then forms of bodybuilding training make the most sense. The bulk of that approach should consist of body part exercises that vary in planes and ranges of motion – a program like my Hardgainer Solution.

Many of the risks involved with weight training after age 50 can be negated with proper programming and correct tactical application during workouts. The risks of training with weights after age 50 are nominal compared to other forms of exercise. Believe it or not, running and jogging tends to create the most injuries compared to any other form of exercise, and this is especially true after age 50.

Hormones and Aging

The human species are really not designed to live into our late 40s and beyond. When human physiology was developing and evolving a couple of million years ago, nobody lived to be any older than about 25, so hormonal decline and its ill effects was not the issue it is today. I want to talk here about three of the main "master hormones" of the body: testosterone, growth hormone, and thyroid hormone. These just happen to be hormones that decline the most with age and tend to have the most pernicious effects on the body—both physique and quality of life—as they decline.

Master hormones are labeled as such because they affect each other and other hormonal systems and biochemical interactions.

Testosterone: Its Function and Benefits

Testosterone is THE master hormone that affects the kind of energy we associate with verve, vitality, exuberance, vigor, and a zest for life. I am not over-emphasizing. There is a reason castration was once used as a medical treatment to calm men down and mellow them out. As testosterone levels diminish in amounts and efficiency as you age, you in essence, function as if being castrated a little bit at a time. Let's talk testosterone's contribution and function.

Everyone is familiar with the sexual function of testosterone. It helps you maintain a healthy libido, and it can help men get and maintain erections. But there is so much more to testosterone and its contributions to a healthy disposition.

Proper testosterone balance, which I consider to be in the high-normal range, helps prevent joint and muscle pain, osteoporosis, and even obesity. Testosterone helps preserve bone mass, reduce fat, and "cellulite." In other words, healthy levels of testosterone help balance your muscle to body fat composition. Plus, healthy levels of testosterone have direct healthy effects on thyroid and leptin. These two hormones themselves in turn have direct effects on a healthy metabolism, as well as a cosmetically beneficial affect on body composition, appetite and weight-control.

Some lesser-known functions of testosterone:

- Reduces the risk of heart disease by protecting the heart and arteries and countering high cholesterol and angina

- Protects major organs like the pancreas, kidneys, and digestive organs

- Helps to tighten and tone the skin

- Protects the thyroid from autoimmune inflammation

- Increases your ability to handle stress, and prevents anxiety, depression and excessive emotionality

- Reinforces memory strength.

As you can see, healthy testosterone levels have a "protective and preventative" effect in many systems of healthy body-regulation. You may be well to consider testosterone as a champion hormone for health and well-being.

The Effects of Low Testosterone (Low-T)

Sooner or later most men will develop a deficiency in testosterone for many reasons. The simple fact is that the tissues and feedback loops that manufacture testosterone just get weaker or wear away as we age.

Everyone is aware of the most common effect of low testosterone in men: having a low or non-existent libido and erectile issues. As most people know, whether through commercials or through real life experience, low levels of testosterone will lead to sexual apathy, weaker erections and ejaculations, and less overall energy and enthusiasm for life. But there is a lot more to the phenomenon of Low-T and its major physiological effects. Having Low-T, doesn't necessarily make you feel bad; but you just don't feel great. You don't feel like your former self for a long period of time, and because the change is so gradual, you chalk it up to other things, like age, stress, lack of sleep, other commitments, etc. You often feel tired, or lazy, and some men experience emotional apathy along with these physical effects. There are of course the physical differences with Low-T. Muscles look softer, and you can put on belly fat more easily.

Testosterone levels peak in our mid-20s, hold relatively steady for another decade or so, and then begin to fall. By the time we're in our late 40s, the human male is figuratively running on hormonal vapors if you will. I know I was by my mid 40s. Interestingly enough, research abounds illustrating that millions of men suffer from low testosterone (hypogonadism) as they age but fewer than 2% seek treatment for it. Yet untreated hypogonadism can lead to fatigue, depression, impotence, low libido, low vitality, fat gain, osteoporosis, and just generally "feeling old."

Furthermore, your creativity can be compromised because your mind is excessively affected by overall somatic fatigue. Cosmetically speaking, the muscles just feel and look more flaccid and soft. And since this particular book is about achieving a better "physique after 50," it bears pointing out the effects that low-T has on the cosmetic appearance of your muscles, skin tone, and overall physique.

But the mental effects of low-T should not be understated either. This book isn't solely about a better Physique after 50. It's also about "Platinum Club Membership" and higher quality of life as we age to 50 and beyond. So, these mental consequences of Low-T need to be highlighted. Some compelling statistics: 90 percent of men diagnosed with low testosterone levels experience nervousness and anxiety. 80 percent of them experience irritability. 56 percent report feeling "off and uncomfortable" and 50 percent report excessive excitability (aka, "edginess.") More than 75 percent experience depression.

Testosterone leads to better more qualitative vitality energy and endurance. Research shows that depression in male patients deficient in testosterone have their depression disappear after they begin using testosterone therapy. There is no doubt that the right amount of circulating testosterone also contributes to a positive mood and disposition;.

As testosterone levels drop, so does the proficiency with which we are able to activate the high threshold motor units for muscular/workout performance. Recruitment of these high threshold motor units is one of the neuromuscular effects of testosterone. As this diminishes as we age - "how much we can lift" becomes less and less. Older trainees have older hormonal and biochemical milieus that diminish optimum stress adaptation and response present in our younger years.

The body's response to training stimulus diminishes as we age.

Because these hormonal and biochemical factors diminish the "response to training" for, people over

50 should not train to failure or exhaustion and not implement training tactics that take muscles beyond normal recovery. If you love weight training, once you're beyond 50, you should NEVER try to lift one-rep maximums (1RM).

Testosterone Benefits For Women

Women's bodies also manufacture testosterone, and like men, it decreases with age, with similar side effects: diminished lean mass, sustainable physical energy, muscle tone, with weight gain, body fat gain, general fatigue, depression, lower sexual interest, and reduced clitoral sensitivity. Lack of testosterone in women is also one of the principle causes of bone loss. Effects of testosterone deficiency can serve as an early-warning sign to women to recognize potential bone loss before it is too late.

Adequate levels of testosterone are important in females as well.

Testosterone is now becoming prescribed more and more for ladies over 40 as part of an overall HRT approach to feeling, functioning, and looking better. Testosterone is also a powerful antidepressant in women, just as it is with men. My female clients who have had testosterone added to their HRT approach, report being happier and more energetic than they have felt in years. The sad part here is that it is still difficult for women to find gynecologists or internal medicine specialists who understand the benefits of testosterone therapy in the pre-, peri-, or post-menopausal female.

Hormone Replacement Therapy (HRT) and The Platinum Club

I am a big proponent of HRT for men *and* women over 50. HRT makes good sense if you want to function with verve and vitality after middle age. Let me clarify that **HRT is not the use of Performance Enhancing Drugs (PED,) or even close to it.** They are entirely different things.

Hormone replacement therapy is about bringing major hormones back in line with normal ranges for someone a bit younger, in their 30s, as an example. PEDs are associated with supra-physiologic doses of drugs designed to enhance athletic performance well beyond 'normal' ranges. That kind of use and abuse carries a lot of risk.

Testosterone treatment for Low-T helps get men to regain lost physical, mental, and emotional vitality and energy. It improves libido and erection quality. It can increase and restore lean tissue mass and strength, strengthen bones, reduce inflammation and decrease the pain of arthritis. It can improve cognition and mood, and improve sleep. (More than 60% of testosterone deficient men also report sleep issues.)

Testosterone treatment gives men (and women) their vitality back.

In my opinion, HRT just makes good sense as we age.

To summarize, when testosterone is deficient, you can feel sluggish and fatigued all day long. You tend to be cloudier in your thinking and less decisive. Low levels of testosterone tend to move your mood toward apathy at first, and then depression. Low levels of testosterone can even lead to disrupted sleep patterns, which in turn lowers testosterone levels even more, leading to a vicious cycle of negative effects in both men and women. There is much more to testosterone than just "muscles, abs, erections, and sex."

Testosterone is a key component to health and well-being for men and women.

If you have any of the signs of testosterone deficiency listed above, see an endocrinologist or internal medicine specialist. I've had many clients to whom I've recommended getting checked out for

HRT, and shortly after going on replacement therapy, they report sleeping and feeling better than they have in months, sometimes years. They often comment "I feel like myself again."

HRT For Women

I am not going to comment a whole lot about HRT for women. Experts vary in their recommendations on HRT for women and ratios of estrogen and progesterone at various stages of menopause, and so forth. Although it's a much more individual thing, I am still a proponent of HRT for women as well.

The reason I discuss more details about testosterone replacement for men and women after 50 is because it is more gender neutral in effects and application than estrogen and progesterone. This doesn't mean women taking HRT will be taking the same doses as men, and suddenly sprouting big muscles and hair in unwanted locations.

Again, I suggest consulting with an endocrinologist or internal medicine specialist if you are a woman and you are considering HRT. Maybe go beyond your family doctor and take the discussion directly to a specialist.

Growth Hormone Considerations

Growth hormone should be considered as the overall "youth hormone."

Growth hormone is responsible for your body maturing through puberty, and serves many other functions as well. It's a reason you can recover so easily from varied physical exertion when you are younger. It's the reason you can pull all-nighters here and there when you are younger and not overly suffer for it. It's the reason you can eat Big Macs and Whoppers and fries when you are younger and not have it negatively impact your cosmetic appearance too much. Growth hormone helps burn fat and sustains leanness. It helps to keep skin tight and youthful.

In terms of physical training, growth hormone aids in recovery by stimulating the secretion of insulin-like growth factor I (IGF-I), the stuff that actually causes repair and recovery to occur. Growth hormone is efficient at cell regeneration and repair and this also includes joint protection as well. This is why younger athletes can compete for so long and so hard.

As we age, growth hormone drops off the same way as testosterone does; it diminishes in both effectiveness and amounts produced. But unlike testosterone, diminished growth hormone affects both genders equally. As we age, both men and women lose the ability to produce GH in response to stimuli that would normally cause an increase in GH levels in a younger adult – like during sleep at night or after intense exercise. There is a linear relationship between GH and IGF-I levels, and therefore a linear relationship between aging and the ability to recover from heavy work. This must be taken into consideration when designing and implementing programs for the over-50 trainee.

Knowing this, we should not be surprised that we gain fat easier, and can't get away with the diet indulgences and indiscretions that we could in our younger years. Diminished growth hormone is directly responsible for what we call "the middle-aged spread," a term used to denote sudden fat gain in the 45 to 55 age range.

I am not ready to endorse GH as part of overall hormone replacement therapy. I don't think the research or the expertise is quite there yet to be able to prescribe growth hormone in the guaranteed healthy ways that overall hormone replacement therapy is. Exogenous growth hormone (prescribed growth hormone, not naturally-secreted) is known to down-regulate thyroid. This can certainly create a very messy hormonal milieu if an expert internal medicine specialist or endocrinologist is not carefully and regularly monitoring blood work.

None of the clients I have coached who are on HRT are taking GH as part of their overall HRT approach to wellness, including me. If all of these youthful effects of growth hormone appeal to you, then you should seek a referral to an internal medicine specialist or endocrinologist and discuss all the details with them.

A Word About Thyroid Hormone

Thyroid hormone may be considered the master energy hormone when it comes to metabolism and autonomic nervous system function. Thyroid hormone *levels* often don't diminish much as we age, but they diminish in usual *effectiveness and function*. This can be tricky, because blood tests can reveal normal circulating levels of thyroid hormone, when the thyroid is underperforming. Hypothyroidism—underperforming thyroid—is one of the most common master hormone issues you can face as you age. Furthermore, if you have had a history of chronic dieting, losing and gaining weight, then your thyroid function is likely to be compromised. Most former female physique competitors I know are on thyroid medications now, and will be for the rest of their lives.

Thyroid issues that arise as you age often masquerade as other ailments entirely.

General symptoms of hypothyroidism include fatigue, lack of focus, feeling cold all the time (especially in the extremities,) fogginess, dizziness, constipation, and of course weight-gain. As with declining levels of testosterone and estrogen/progesterone in women, many people just chalk this up to being a consequence of aging.

The thyroid hormone replacement drug Synthroid® (levothyroxine), used for underactive thyroids or post-thyroidectomy, is in the top three most-prescribed medications in North America. Anywhere from 70 to 100 million people take the medication. And yet thyroid hormone is still likely being under-prescribed as most people live unknowingly with the effects of thyroid problems.

Overactive thyroid – known as hyperthyroidism – can mask as jitteriness, ADD, heart arrhythmias, muscle weakness (just like with hypothyroid), anxiety, depression, apathy, and even osteoporosis. As many as 10 percent of adults age 50 and older have some form of thyroid disorder.

Thyroid replacement medication is safe and effective. My ex-wife has been taking Synthroid for an under-active thyroid for over 40 years now, and she is probably the most active and energetic person I know. I've been taking Synthroid® myself for well over a decade and I have no issues at all.

Once thyroid malfunction is being medically treated, then issues related to thyroid are no longer a problem.

After age 40, you should be getting regular blood tests done, and regular thyroid function tests as part of this overall blood work.

What this all means for Physique After 50

What am I illustrating above are the realities of the more major hormonal and biochemical changes that come with aging. And they tend to come quicker and be more pronounced around age 50 and onward.

A change in thyroid combined with decreased testosterone, menopause in women, decreased growth hormone in men and women, can together compound how "old" actually feel inside. This can add to the risks for poor joint health, risk of disease, risk of deteriorating mental health, and more. To accept it as a part of aging simply makes no sense to me when you can choose to do something about it.

It is also true that if you take better care of your body, then your body will take better care of you than you may realize.

Weight training keeps the hormone stimulus-response and biochemical systems functioning much better and deteriorating much less slowly, even though deterioration is inevitable.

I suggest you check into HRT, and keep getting your blood checked after age 50 for signs of hormonal change and deterioration. A little hormonal restoration will keep you feeling better and enhance the quality of your life. When combined with resistance training, you will also enhance the quality of your appearance and how you feel.

Chapter 2.

What Form of Training is Best?

Body part resistance training, with weights and other resistance equipment, stands out above all the rest when it comes to working out for people over 50. It helps you to continually recharge and offset the effects of aging. Aside from what should be its obvious benefits for muscles and posture, it makes the most sense and is the better exercise choice for metabolism, bone, and joint health. It's just better all around. I've summarized the benefits below.

Metabolism. Some kind of exercise is going to be necessary to offset your slowing metabolism. A slower metabolism leads to weight-gain and sluggishness. Weight training has the greatest effects in terms of optimizing metabolism, because it optimizes lean tissue gain and retention.

Bone health. Bone health becomes more and more important as you age. Weight-bearing exercise is going to benefit your bones. Resistance training will also help you to become more mobile.

Joint health. Regular resistance training strengthens muscles surrounding the joint, thereby adding support. The right kind of resistance training will also help to offset varying kinds of painful inflammation. Weaker, atrophied muscles make joints more susceptible to overuse injuries and injuries in general. By exercising specific muscles through a full range of motion, the muscles become more mobile and less constricted. This makes basic every day functions easier.

There are all kinds of reasons to work out with weights and resistance train after age 50. It boils down to one word really – "prevention." Working out with weights after age 50 helps you offset the effects of sarcopenia and it is the best form of preventative exercise for the years to come. It has important cosmetic as well. You can still sculpt a physique after age 50. The cosmetic benefits become self-motivating as people take notice, comment, and ask what kind of exercise you do. Ask any bodybuilder: this type of reinforcement helps keep you going back to the gym.

I've been weight training and living the fitness lifestyle in general for many years, and more recently the Physique After 50 body part training lifestyle. I've been asked twice in the last month to show someone my ID because they couldn't believe that I was turning 55 years young. Another gentleman stopped me in the gym to tell me how motivating it is for him to watch me work out. Recently, a young client in his 30s flew into town to train with me and learn, After several days of training with me he said, "Man, you still got it Coach." Those kinds of comments are very motivating, no matter whom you are. And at any age, we should gather our motivations from as many sources as we can. The point here is I can keep up without trying to keep up, because of the lifestyle I live, and the kind of training that I do, keeps me looking younger and functioning more youthfully.

What exactly is "Body Part Resistance Training"?

Body part resistance training is more or less traditional bodybuilding training. This means training all the general muscles of the body specifically, in an isolated way, with weights, or other type of resistance, such as elastic tubing, cables, or your own bodyweight.

Body part bodybuilding training means resistance training with a focus on "surfing the strength curve" of repetitions while doing various exercises for each body part. The phrase "surfing the strength curve" itself means utilizing a *wide range of repetition ranges* within a workout or overall workout program.

This type of training can also be referred to as "strength-density-training," or "Innervation Training Methodology." Typically, advanced bodybuilders tend to train one specific body part per workout. So their training week might look like something as simple as this breakdown: Day One: Chest, - Day Two: Back, - Day Three: Shoulders, - Day Four: Arms (biceps and triceps), - Day Five: Legs – followed by a day or two off. Within each session, they will do anywhere from three to six exercises for that target muscle group, and do anywhere from three to six sets per exercise for anywhere from five to 20 reps, typically. And of course this approach can vary.

I am not suggesting someone simply take up this advanced bodybuilding approach. There are better approaches for the over-50 age group. For instance, my *Hardgainer Solution* program applies a body part approach to a whole body workout. In Hardgainer Solution, I say directly that trainees over 50 years of age would definitely be considered "hardgainers."

If you are someone over 50, unless you compete in some kind of very specific athletic event, then the various forms of functional training and Olympic lifts with barbells are simply unnecessary and very high-risk forms of training for you in general. Both of these types of training can be very ballistic, subjecting the joints to shocking levels of force. Body part training is far gentler and safer. Your workout regimen has to be smarter after age 50. This means excluding as much injury risk and joint trauma as possible in your resistance training approach. Traditional body part training does that very thing.

A traditional bodybuilding body part training approach makes the most sense for sustainable exercise regimens after age 50.

As I was compiling my notes for this project, an older gentleman in the gym asked me this very important and pertinent question,, "What is more important after age 50, cardio or resistance training?" I'm glad he asked. The question reminded me of the stale fitness-related myths that continue among consumers. Most people still carry this untrue and naïve notion that aerobic/cardio activity is better and safer for you than weight training. Moreover, most uninformed consumers still believe that aerobic training is better for weight-control and fat loss. None of these are true, and even more untrue for people over 50.

We've already discussed how metabolism slows

with age, and it becomes quite noticeable starting as early as age 35 (in women especially.) Weight training and regular exercise can slow these effects to be sure. Exercise to engage muscle mass – as in body part training – keeps metabolism as optimized and robust as possible. Contrary to popular belief, "cardio" exercise has little to no effect on retarding the slow-down of metabolism, and if over-used can make it worse through loss of lean muscle mass. Cardio does not offset sarcopenia whereas weight training does.

Walking may be the ultimate form of non-resistance exercise after age 50. Jogging and running is ill advised because of the pounding on knees and alignment issues with hips and low back. Running and jogging have always been higher risk of injury activities than weight training. Walking is safe, it's weight bearing, and it doesn't require equipment or a special environment. I walk outside after my workouts from late February till November. I don't recommend the use weights when walking for fitness. Hand weights can cause shoulder pain, alignment issues, back issues, elbow or wrist issues. Ankle weights can cause knee strain and also create alignment issues. Just walk faster if you want to make walking harder.

Too many people make the mistake of getting caught-up in quantifying calorie burning in exercise.

This is a mistake and it's misleading. The calorie-burning nature of a workout should take a distant second place to metabolic optimization effects. Those metabolic effects will play out over the long term, not just within the workout itself. Especially if you are over 50, resistance training makes better sense than worrying about calorie-burning activities, like elliptical or treadclimber machines, or boot camp classes, which have some cardio-pulmonary benefit, but do not sculpt physique nor battle sarcopenia. Activities like boot camp classes are dangerous for people over 50.

After considering all the pros and cons, body part, "bodybuilding" training—properly implemented—still makes the most sense for members of the Platinum club in terms of joint health and protection, programming, recovery and systemic benefit.

This Is NOT Pure Strength Training

Pure strength training most often refers to the powerlifts: barbell bench press, squat, and deadlift, and training to achieve a One Rep Maximum (1RM.) Body part and strength training are two very different kinds of weight training. Trainees 50 and older may want to avoid these focus barbell lifts. Be aware that experts on aging often equate all resistance training to 'strength training,' a mistake that can be quite misleading if taken literally.

I want to be very specific here so that people understand some major differences in training methods. I use a broad based terms like "resistance training" and "weight training" deliberately to avoid using the term "strength training." While resistance training and weight training will indeed make you stronger, this is not what is meant by the term "strength training." When experts in our industry (the iron game) use the term "strength training," they are almost always referring to what is called "limit strength training." That form of training is all about lifting more weight. And it is also almost always a focus on lifting more weight in the barbell squat, bench press, and deadlift. Often they include movements like barbell power cleans, and chin-ups.

They cling to "how much you lift" as the main indicator for workout performance. Both these things focus on what I call "external cues." In the aging body, this is not conducive to long-term sustainability, injury prevention or joint health.

The wise sculpted physique approach focuses on neither specific "magic barbell exercises," nor how much you lift.

The "sculpted physique" approach is to focus on the muscle, and how it feels. This is what I call an "internal cue." Internal cues keep you connected to the biofeedback of your working muscles. These strength experts, even as they themselves age, still hold onto the notion that "the weights work the muscles" – an external cue emphasis.

So, I will repeat well-known Abel-isms which is even more imperative for the over 50 trainee:

"Train the muscle not the movement."

Experts who are about pure strength training, almost without exception, associate only barbell work and lifting loads to that equation. This is a mistake when considering the over-50 trainee. For example, barbell training and strength expert Mark Rippetoe—whose knowledge I respect a great deal—has said in more than one of his books that, now that he is in his 50s, his training really hurts and causes him pain. Rippetoe said, "But lots of master's lifters — and maybe most of us — train hurt. It's either that or not train at all, so we train hurt."

I actually can't believe he said that! Taken to its logical conclusion, training hurt eventually leads to training being physically impossible, regardless of pain tolerance; and that means accepting a sedentary lifestyle at some point in the future.

Rippetoe's comment reflects the paradigm blindness of strength experts. Many of these strength experts constantly disparage and belittle bodybuilders and their training, and this bias blinds them to its benefits. Rippetoe himself explains quite well the trauma of barbell bench presses in relation to the shoulder joint.

He makes that statement within a very limited and biased context, because he can't let go of thinking that barbell training and the powerlifting exercises are the "best" forms of training, even when that form of training itself is what is causing and exacerbating the pain.

If these experts gave dumbbells and body part training focused on "training the muscle, not the movement" an honest try, they might enjoy weight training more, experience far less pain, and get more out of their workouts and exercise regimens. Rippetoe himself also made this statement: "The longer I stay in this business, the less fond I become of the bench press." And yet he didn't follow that statement up with recommendations for dumbbell bench press or incline dumbbell work, or other body part exercises and orientations.

All the above leads me to using the terms "resistance training" and "weight training" and body part training, instead of lumping all this terminology together under a misleading term "strength training." The benefits of the bodybuilding body part training methodology for trainees over 50 far outweigh the benefits of any other form of exercise – and especially outweigh the risks and wear and tear of pure strength training.

Special Training Caveats to Consider

Exercise, and sports activities of all kinds, carries risk of injury, at any age. It surprises most people to learn that injuries from running and jogging rank the highest in terms of types of exercise causing injury. Weight training actually ranks among the lowest risk forms of exercise, but it still must be done right. For our age group, the risk of injury, or training-induced chronic conditions, increases because of age, not because of the activity itself.

The potential for injuries, or nagging aches and pains that limit your training, must be managed carefully for this reason. However, training hard enough to force progress yet light enough to avoid injuries, can be a difficult balancing act. You can still make progress, or I wouldn't be writing this project. How much progress you can make depends on what you do based on how advanced you are with your training. Developing and sculpting a physique after

50 can be challenging, but that is what also makes it fun and intriguing.

You want to make sure that you work your muscles efficiently. The key here is to not overstress the joints at the same time. You want to eliminate exercises that are dangerous, or that subject the joints to intense and sudden shock. You want to avoid harsh jarring motions and a lot of ballistic movements, such as plyometric work (jumping, hopping, bounding, etc.) Finally, you want to minimize, but not necessarily eliminate compressive forces on the spine. My 6 Day PA50 is a program that does this. The beginner version is safe and protective. I have a list of exercises and tactical approaches in a later section that outline in greater detail what to do, what *not* to do and the like. But first, I want to outline just a few more types of training to avoid and why.

As I outlined above already, many strength experts – the ones who get the most attention on industry websites—like to glorify the powerlifts, and this emphasis trickles down to gym floor influences. But for the 50-plus age demographic and for the purpose of cosmetic physique enhancement and development, the **bench press** is just another exercise. There's nothing special about it. For members of the Platinum club, the bench press should be done with dumbbells instead of barbells.

DB use facilitates a more effective and safer line of action for the pectorals, with less shoulder and elbow joint strain, and leads to better muscle fiber recruitment.

Barbell bench presses and barbell inclines after age 45 scare me. The rigid bar is tough on the shoulder capsule and the rotator cuffs. This can lead to chronic pain, inflammation, range of motion (ROM) restriction and injury if it goes on too long. DBs are the way to go for these movements if you are over age 45 or so.

If you have any low back issues, you should best avoid **barbell back squats** as well. While the squat motion is fine and an essential part of most viable training programs, squats do not have to be done in a way that creates as much spinal compression as barbell back squats do. Spinal compression risks aside, barbell back squats put the shoulder joint in a very uncomfortable position as well.

The **barbell deadlift** shouldn't be done at all if you are over 50, although the RDL version has some value. Barbell deadlifts would be used minimally, if at all, in a body part program for Platinum Club members. In fact, I don't have the barbell deadlift anywhere in my Hardgainer Solution. Now, many strength experts, powerlifters and exercise professionals may argue with me on this point. There are likely many trainees over 50 doing barbell deadlifts. So be it. I say the risk is not worth the reward, and for cosmetic physique enhancement after 50, the deadlift simply doesn't offer very much value.

Let me add this: Just as DB bench press is a safer alternative to barbell bench press for Physique After 50 trainees, the same can be true for DB squats and DB deadlifts, although to a lesser degree. If you do squats and deadlifts with DBs – that is with DBs hanging at your side, and not on your shoulders – then you can still reap the kinetic chain and metabolic effects of these two movements with minimal spinal compression forces. You will minimize injury risk and joint trauma by eliminating the barbell variations, or by switching the DB variations with DBs hanging at the side of each leg to execute the movements.

Moving away from specific exercises for a bit, I would also like to comment on various forms of exercise as well; specifically "boot camps," "group fitness" classes, and branded, Workout Of the Day (aka WOD) programs (e.g., CrossFit®) that emphasize hard work without regard for exhaustion or injury.

Very often these one-size-fits-all approaches incorporate a lot of plyometric work and jumping around, with everyone encouraged to train at the same pace and same level of intensity. Unless you are in exceptional physical condition already, then this is not a good idea if you are over 50 and trying to protect your joints. And unless the class is entirely composed of people over 50 like yourself, you would be wise to avoid them. You also need to know that these types of classes are not going to lead to any kind of real physique-sculpting either.

Exercise has to be about more than just burning off calories, especially once you are over 50.

Finally, getting it right with 'Physique After 50' means 'training your age.' You can't work out like younger people do, and it's a mistake to think you can. Do not try to keep up with younger trainees. And do not try to work out the way you did when *you* were younger. Sylvester Stallone comes to mind as an example. Stallone was still training his body, not his age, as he got older. That led him to some serious training-related injuries. Stallone tore his pec, and then had other issues that messed up his physique cosmetically. He has since modified his training to suit his age, but not before he paid a serious price with injury and bodily disfigurement from doing workouts that did not take his age into consideration.

Like it or not, after age 50, you must "train your age."

That is great advice for staying healthy, injury-free, and able to sustain working out as a lifestyle.

Chapter 3.

Forget About It

For the sake of argument, let's employ the catch phrase **"Forget About It"** for training-related things you should leave in the rear-view mirror.

"Forget About It" is not absolute. It is a general statement of priorities, except when I point them out as things to "never" do. Some of what you'll see below is restated in this section for special emphasis. I've added headings that allow you to reference this section often as you review your training efforts and workouts.

Forget about training to failure

Only athletes with very high thresholds of work capacity from decades of training should train to failure. And even then this would be on a limited basis. If you see someone with a jacked-up, massive physique training to failure, they are probably on PEDs, which enhance their workout abilities and recovery capacity. Training to failure taps into recovery needs beyond what the body can adequately recover from in a reasonable time frame. Going "all out" after age 50 is likely to lead to burnout or even injury. Always leaving a few reps in the tank short of failure is a good rule to abide by when training for a sculpted and balanced physique after 50.

Training should not burn you out; it should invigorate you.

Forget about barbell pressing movements

I am specifically referring to barbell bench press, and barbell military press (shoulder press,) both in front or behind the head. These movements just accelerate joint trauma on the shoulder, no matter how safely they are performed. You can get just as much positive effect or better, by using either DB variations of these movements, or machine and cable variations as well. Barbells are just too rigid in creating fixed positions in pressing movements. And overtime this can really adversely impact the shoulder joint.

Forget about barbell deadlifts (especially if spinal compression is an issue)

As I stated above, the barbell deadlift itself really doesn't add much value in terms of targeted body part training for creating a balanced physique, and is best avoided for any older trainee with even a hint of low back issues. The DB version is still fine, but also not necessary. In the DB version, the DBs hang at your sides and not in front, offsetting a lot of spinal compression, while still offering the kinetic chain expression of ground forces through the lift's completion.

While the RDL deadlift may have some value, the Barbell Sumo deadlift really has no value at all for better Physique After 50. The BB Sumo Deadlift is a lifting technique that some lifters find offers them better leverage. Given that all forms of deadlifts have a higher injury risk, the BB Sumo deadlift really is a movement you can completely forget about when it comes to training for a better Physique After 50.

Forget about explosive stuff and plyometrics

To protect the joints, sudden impact exercises and jarring motions such as explosive push-ups, squat jumps, and other plyo drills with resistance, should be avoided. Perhaps more to the point, these movements just are not necessary to build a physique. They are not worth the risk to joint health.

Forget about Barbell Olympic Lifts

The snatch lift, the clean and jerk, and barbell power cleans can be dangerous moves in general. The barbell power clean is particularly hard on the shoulder joints, elbows and wrists. It is also a very technical lift that can lead to injury if it is not done properly. DB versions and variations of these lifts still offer some value and can be used in a safer way with less trauma to the joints.

But they still are not necessary exercises to developing a physique after 50. DB variations of Olympic lifts are included in some of my workout plans, but not in the plans I prescribe for Physique After 50. You can forget about these if your goal is sculpting a better physique after 50, and especially if you have limited-to-no prior lifting experience with these technical lifts.

Forget about pull ups, muscle ups, and kipping chin-ups

These movements are very popular in the CrossFit training world. But they are also very hard on the joints, and are also unnecessary when training for a sculpted physique. These movements do not target and overload a single body part very effectively. Some people may like to do chin-ups. They are fine for part of a back workout protocol, if you can do them pain-free and perform them smoothly and effectively from the first rep. There is nothing magical about being able to do chin-ups or pull-ups. But the kipping chin-up, so popular in the CrossFit world, should be avoided.

Forget About Battling Ropes

This is a particularly nasty exercise that invites trauma to the shoulder joint and adds no value. I see no reason why this exercise should ever be included in a program for any trainee over 50. Frankly, I am not fond of "battling ropes" for any trainee. Recently I witnessed a personal trainer getting a man to do the battling ropes exercise. This man was is in his 60s and he was obviously fairly new to training. While doing the battling ropes it was clear he already had shoulder joint issues especially on one side. The whole thing looked incredibly awkward and painful, and instead of stopping him from doing the exercise, the trainer told the man not to worry and that he would get used to it. The man ended up holding one arm a few minutes later as if it was in a sling, no doubt caused by battling ropes.

Forget about overstating abs training

When I say forget about abs training, I mean leaving out special emphasis on abs and core training as a focus all its own. What I am talking about here is to not over-emphasize abs work by doing too much of it as in a separate workout, or overloading abs work at the end of a workout. There is seldom a reason for someone over 50 to be isolating abs training with emphasis. Doing so can lead to all kinds of imbalance issues and make back and abs areas susceptible to injury. In some programs, it may not be necessary at all. For example, there is no abs training at all in the beginner program supplied with this project.

Forget about forced reps

This is a lifting technique used by mostly by the more hardcore trainees in the bodybuilding world. Forced reps rely on a partner to help you do more reps of an exercise after you have already reached repetition failure on your own. This was a bad idea when it first became popular and it's a bad idea now. But it's an especially bad idea for a trainee over 50. A forced rep by its very name suggests you are already tapping into your recovery ability. You are forcing your muscles to do more repetitions of an exercise after the muscles have already reached failure. Because recovery between workouts is such an important concern for any trainee over 50, forced reps is one of those hardcore techniques that you need to forget about completely.

Forget about heavy negatives

This is another hardcore technique that is best forgotten. But it's especially crucial to avoid if you are over 50. Heavy negatives is an old training technique where you overload the bar with more weight than you can lift concentrically, then slowly lower the bar in the eccentric phase of an exercise (usually something like bench press,) and then a training partner helps you lift the weight back to the starting position for several repetitions. "Negatives" are often done at the end of a training set without the "heavy" emphasis, where they become another sort of forced reps variation. Doing "negatives" in training is based on research that shows that muscles can handle a lot more weight and are stronger eccentrically than they can lift concentrically. This somehow carried over into gym lore as a useful training tactic. Well, it's not. It's one of those leftover faulty ideas from a bygone era. Doing heavy negatives has no place in any program, but something you should forget about completely, and never do, if you are over 50.

Forget about max lifts

Developing and sculpting a physique at any age has never been about max lifts, as in seeing how much you can bench press for one repetition. Max lift training is only about massaging your ego. There is added danger in training to see how much you can lift one time in any of the major lifts. This tends to also put a lot of unnecessary stress on the joints, which we are trying to avoid in the over 50 trainee. Now, if someone is powerlifting safely over 50, more power to them. But for the trainee seeking fitness and a more cosmetically appealing physique after age 50, max lifts are useless, and you need to forget about them.

Forget about tempo training

This is something you are likely to hear from personal trainers, and it is a particular pet peeve of mine. Tempo training is where you are instructed to count on the concentric phase of a rep, then the eccentric phase of a rep, and sometimes even in the static phase of a set between reps. It's a lot of hyped-up nonsense that doesn't offer any real value. It is one of the many things we label as "an illusion of control."

You should be learning how to concentrate and feel the targeted muscles working. Counting just distracts you from that, because you are thinking about numbers, instead of about how your muscles feel. Furthermore, many exercises are not designed for a slower eccentric phase. Learning the pumping cadence of executing reps is the proper way to perform traditional bodybuilding/body part training. I've trained pros, and trained *with* top pros for most of my career, and none of them used "tempo" training. If you watch the movie "Pumping Iron" you will see that NO ONE training in this movie uses it either. Tempo training is just more modern made-up madness that adds more confusion than it does value. Forget about it!

Forget about cardio

A lot of people won't like that comment. But people who don't like that comment are not looking at it objectively from the purely physiological standpoint. Too many misinformed trainees get stuck in this notion of cardio as "fat burning" activity. This is a misinterpretation of the facts. When you are over 50, too much cardio is a tissue destroying activity, the last thing you want from exercise when you are trying to offset the ravages of sarcopenia.

A little cardio activity isn't going to be enough to burn much fat anyway, and furthermore, a lot of cardio activity will likely invite overuse injuries and conditions in those over 50.

Now, of course there are exceptions, as there always are. The exception here is that if you just enjoy aerobic and cardio activity for cardiovascular effects, then do it, as in walking, power walking, or even cycling, but not running, jogging, or sprinting. Walking is a great choice for aerobic activity, especially if you can do it outside. Another exception would be for those who are very overweight, for whom some walking or cycling makes sense from an overall conditioning standpoint. But still, no running, jogging or sprinting.

If you think you are going to lose fat in all the right areas from cardio activity, you do need to forget about it. So when I say, "forget about cardio," what I really mean is:

1) Forget about cardio as a primary exercise if you are trying to change your physique

2) Forget about cardio as your primary exercise for burning fat

3) Forget about cardio as your primary exercise to offset the effects of sarcopenia.

Forget about pre-, peri-, and post-training meal planning

If you are reading this book, you likely are not currently a world class athlete training for hours per day at maximum work capacity; so, pre-, peri, and post-training meal tactics do not apply. The fitness industry likes to take certain things like this – things that apply in a very specific and limited context – and generalize so that they can sell supplements to more people. Those who are pushing the limits of their bodies *for competitive purposes* plan meals around workouts. If you are training for a better-developed, sculpted Physique After 50, then you should be deliberately *under-training* and not ever maxing out your body's recovery capacity by pushing it to its limits. All you really need to concentrate on is eating balanced meals throughout the day; meals composed of healthy whole, unprocessed foods. Do not buy into industry hype when it comes to special drinks or concoctions to consume before, during, or after training. This simply does not apply to the over 50 trainee, so you can forget about it.

Chapter 4.

Crucial Considerations

I call this section "crucial considerations" for a reason. It is a general checklist of preventative measures for you to follow when training after age 50. The list takes into account the realities about our aging bodies.

No doubt about it, as we age and get into our 50s, the risk of injury goes up, including minor injuries occurring outside the exercise regimen, and more serious injuries from exercise itself.

The preventative and "prehab" work described here become important considerations for this demographic.

Proper Programming

Sound programming simply makes sense at any age, but even more so after age 50.

From the get-go, you should invest in some kind of real training "program" to follow. It also helps if you invest in programs that are designed specifically for you, that suit your age and lifestyle. The PA50 programs provided here are designed for this purpose, as is my Hardgainer Solution Program.

I would *not* advise boot camp classes not aimed specifically at an over 50 age group. I cannot recommend CrossFit® either.

Warm-ups

By this point, I hope you are convinced that, in general, traditional bodybuilding/body part training is the way to enhance a Physique After 50. The joints must be prepared for training single joint and multi-joint (compound) exercises when performed with resistance and in various planes and ranges of motion. Far too many trainees of all ages give scant attention to proper warm-ups for weight training workouts. This is never a good idea at any age. While you may be able to get away with it in your younger years, proper warm-ups for working out become "crucial considerations" for the Physique After 50 demographic.

It is therefore imperative to warm up the major joints—hips, knees, low back and shoulders—before every single workout. These warm-ups need to be considered from this general approach, as well as a more precise, targeted warm-up for the specific workout about to be performed. Over the course of the last six to seven years, I developed a very precise warm-up sequence to support any kind of weight training bodybuilding training workouts. This daily workout warm-up combines what we call GPP (General Preparation Phase,) with what I call "Physical Rehearsal," which is targeting a warm-up toward the specific training workout you are about to undertake. This warm-up regimen accomplishes both without being too different workout to workout. Let me explain GPP and Physical Rehearsal.

GPP (General Preparation Phase)

Experts once agreed that proper warm-up for weight training meant sitting on a bike or walking on a treadmill to warm up. These faulty notions have been rightly replaced by a more sound approach. GPP refers to loosening and warming up the major joints of the body so that the muscles will also respond accordingly with less restricted range of motion.

I have tailored my warm-up sequence for the Physique After 50 trainee to insure constant warm-up and appropriate mobility for the shoulders, knees, hips, low back, without getting overwhelmed with unnecessary complication.

The GPP part of a workout should last no more than five to seven minutes. It consists of:

- Gentle arm swings in various directions for shoulders
- Light tubing pull-aparts also for shoulders/scapula
- Gentle twisting and reaching for the core, waist and low back
- The reach lunge sequence for low back and lower body, and
- "Unloading" the knees by offsetting bodyweight and gently settling into the full squat position.

Unloading the knees is a particularly unique warm-up exercise I developed, that is now catching on everywhere. I want to stress that you should *always* 'unload the knees' as part of every warm-up session, whether you are training legs or not.

Physical Rehearsal

Physical rehearsal refers to two elements of warming up. First, it refers to doing the GPP for the first joint complex that will be the focus on the workout. If your first exercise of the day is going to be an upper body exercise, then you will do the GPP upper body sequence first. You can just continue the lower body sequence GPP between sets of your first exercise. Or, if your first exercise is a complex and it is going to combine an upper body exercise with a lower body exercise—as is often the case in my HGS program – then you will complete the whole GPP sequence before seguing to "physical rehearsal" sets.

An easy definition of physical rehearsal is doing light, slow and easy sets of the first exercise for that particular workout day. For example, if today has a leg focus, beginning with leg press, then you would do your lower body GPP first, followed by a few light, slow sets of the leg press. This allows you to gradually warm up the specific area, and then progress through light sets, on into your "work sets."

Rotator Cuff Exercises

Like unloading the knees, some mild rotator cuff work should be done at least twice a week, or as often as every single training session. I recommend doing the rotator cuff exercises at, or near, the end of the workout. This saved me from shoulder replacement surgery. I progressed from doing overhead presses in pain with 25 lb. DBs, to 70 lb. DBs, more or less pain-free.

Before doing these simple internal and external rotator cuff exercises I had received the maximum amount of cortisone injections allowed, and they didn't help much at all. After about six weeks of doing these simple rotator cuff exercises at the end of my training sessions every day, my pain decreased and my strength and performance increased. These exercises are very easy to do and don't take much time. So if you have any shoulder area issues at all, these rotator cuff exercises are a must. I recommend doing them anyway for shoulder health after age 50, even if only for a couple sets of 10-15 reps at the end of an exercise session.

Spinal Compression Exercises

If you have a history of back issues, after 50 is not the time to try new exercises that compress the spine a lot, or produce inordinate amounts of lower lumbar strain. Therefore normal barbell deadlifts and barbell squats are not my recommended exercise choices for trainees over 50. Dumbbell versions—where the DBs hang at your sides—are much safer to perform and still offer a similar training effect. Again, safety and prevention are key considerations for the over 50 trainee.

Now, having said this, I know there are many trainees out there who are over 50 and who can still do these exercises without much risk, and that is fine. Most of them have decades of lifting experience behind them. So I am not addressed them with this particular over-to "crucial consideration." However, I do have many clients, current and former, who like me, have hurt their lower backs at some point in their training career. So for them I absolutely advise avoiding these barbell movements, or any unnecessary lower lumbar strain in training. For example, right now I have one client who just turned 40 years old. He competed for years and even won Nationals in bodybuilding. But he tweaked his back a while ago, so now he avoids barbell bent rows, barbell deadlifts, and barbell squats, and only uses DB variations as I have instructed him. He remains injury-free as a result. So, if you have any history of lower back issues at all, then it is a "crucial consideration" to minimize spinal compression, or lower lumbar-bearing loads.

Biofeedback

Simply put, biofeedback is what your body tells you. But it is also what your body is *not* telling you. An everyday example of biofeedback would be hunger. Hunger tells you that your body wants or needs food, but it never tells you to *over*-eat – not even if you've missed a previous meal.

It takes practice to read biofeedback correctly because it can be misinterpreted. Using our hunger example, responding correctly might be to question if the previous meal was sufficient to maintain a "tolerable hunger," where an incorrect response might be to give in to a craving, or to confuse a hunger with a craving to begin with. (Hunger is physiological. Cravings are psychological.)

So, knowledge and experience, gained through practice, becomes an important component for interpreting, and responding to, your biofeedback. Biofeedback is listening to your body, then supporting it and nurturing it nutritionally, emotionally, and mentally. A follow-up book to PA50 will go into greater detail on this.

As you age, *correctly and appropriately* reading and responding to your own intra-workout biofeedback, and biofeedback in general, becomes more important than ever for your health and your well-being.

Let's get practical with some examples, beginning with what biofeedback is *not*.

Take workouts for instance. Biofeedback is *not about* watching a clock between sets. And it's not about basing the start of your next set on a wrist-worn heart rate monitor.

In terms of intra-workout biofeedback, a helpful technique to help train you to read biofeedback is to ask yourself questions during the course of your workout (intra-workout), or even "micro-questions" during the course of a set. , Useful questions might include:

- How did that rep or set *feel*? Did that hurt in the wrong way? Was the weight too light, or too heavy in comparison to the targeted rep range? How many more reps could I have done? In PA50, remember we don't train to failure on any set. (No rep or set should hurt in your joints. You shouldn't be feeling stabbing, sharp pains in your muscles. Midway through a high-rep set, you may begin to feel that lactic acid "burn," which is normal. You should feel like you could have done another rep or three.)

- How about oxygen debt? Was I too out of breath after that set? Did I have to sit down to rest between sets?

- Did I achieve a pump? (If not, and you did everything right, it could signal a dietary consideration.)

- Did I leave the gym invigorated, or exhausted?

Biofeedback requires that you are always willing to accept to what your body is telling you. The more experienced you are, the better you become at reading biofeedback. But you must practice doing so. I have clients that have been with me for more than a decade and they still run their biofeedback past me, just to be sure. It's not always clear-cut. If you're new to weight training, this is where a Coach can help. Now, you just have to be very, very cautious in coach selection. There are many more know-nothing personal trainers than there are true Coaches (capital C) who truly know what they're doing, and fewer still who know a thing about biofeedback, pay attention to it, and monitor it.

Chapter 5.

Safety and Injury Prevention

Machines are your friend

This is the exact opposite of early years of training when you are correctly advised to compose most of your training of barbells and dumbbells. But after age 50, machines are your friends. Machines offer a controlled plane of motion and less strain on the joints. While machines should not necessarily compose the majority of the exercises in your routine, they now become a smart choice to include in your training sessions.

Dumbbell-focused training

Most of your workouts should consist of DB-focused movements and exercises – even if they mimic barbell movements: flat or incline DB press for chest, bent DB rows, DB Squats and DB Deadlifts, with DBs hanging at your sides. Due to their versatility and safety, most workouts in the PA50 program will be composed of dumbbells and machines, combined in an intelligent way.

Intra- and Inter-Workout Recovery Considerations

This is a crucial consideration that is often ignored since we seem to be going through a pop-culture phase where training is being designed more and more to pound the body into the ground. As I said in my Hardgainer Solution book, training pace must be sustainable long-term.

Intra-workout recovery. When training for sculpting a physique after 50, very low oxygen debt signals proper pace. Once you begin your workout, your breathing can be labored, but you should never be panting or entirely out of breath. Now, high repetition leg work is going to produce a marked oxygen debt post-set; and there are other exceptions. But *intra*-workout recovery means establishing a sustainable training pace, so that you can train more often and not burn out. And remember, those over 50 should never train to failure on any exercise.

Inter-workout recovery. Never training to failure on any exercise alone should allow muscles to recover between workouts, if you are doing a well-designed program like PA50. If you train at a sustainable pace, and you do not train your muscles to failure on any exercise, then your *inter*-workout recovery should be fine. Never push yourself to your maximum training capacity.

The "Pumping Cadence"

I have discussed this pumping cadence a lot lately in my articles and Podcasts. If you agree that traditional bodybuilding/body part training is the way to go for physique transformation after age 50, then you should agree with the concept of "the pumping cadence." Once reps increase above five or six, then it's a "pumping" kind of cadence you should be shooting for when executing your reps within a workout. For health, for performance, for cosmetic results, and for training longevity, learning how to produce a pumping cadence when doing your exercises is highly recommended. You learn this cadence more by *"feel"* than anything else.

There is no better tool for the learning the pumping cadence than watching the documentary *Pumping Iron* several times, even if you just skip to the training sequences.

All this new age nonsense of personal trainer "tempo training" is completely misguided. You should *feel* your reps when training, not measure them with silly tempos. Concentrate on the muscles you're working, instead of counting.

You won't need a "spotter" when in pumping cadence. If you ever think you need "a spotter" to perform an exercise, then the weight you are using is too heavy. After 50, you never need to be pushing loads so heavy that you need a spotter.

Chapter 6.

Lifestyle

After decades coaching people into physique transformation, it still amazes me how people tend to overlook the elements of lifestyle that make or break it. Many set a goal to take better care of themselves, and to transform themselves from the outside-in. Then they get all caught up in incidental elements of the process. They overlook the most fundamental aspect that make sustainable physique transformation possible, and that is lifestyle consideration.

Lifestyle—composed of things like time and stress management, mindset, attitude, sleep patterns, meal times—lays a foundation that supports all these other training-related pursuits. If you don't have the right lifestyle and the right mindset, then a fitness program is never going to work for long.

So in this section, we are going to explore some of

the most important elements of lifestyle considerations that you need to take charge of, if you ever hope to accomplish and sustain a physique transformation after age 50.

Time and Stress Management

It takes some sort of structure in your life to be able to consistently work out after age 50. Older trainees have other things going on in life. So this requires structure *and* organization.

Older trainees who look great are usually high-functioning people, who tend to be responsible, structured, and daring, with a strong work ethic, intelligence, determination, and character. It's common for people of all ages to look for magic programs. But especially in the Platinum Club – elements of character, routine, and structure become vitally important. You have to be better than ever before at managing your time, including setting regular meal times and workout times.

Many people, especially in their early 50s can have a lot family stresses. Many in our age group often become caught in a "care-giving" matrix, taking care of so many people that they lose the time, energy and space to take care of themselves. I have more than a few male and female clients trapped in this care-giving matrix, caring for aging parents, children and maybe even grandchildren. On top of this you still likely have your own jobs, careers, and spouses to consider. This leads to feeling trapped in a hamster wheel of unpredictability.

There is no easy solution to the care-giving matrix. However, most experts agree that, at any age as an adult, prioritizing self-care makes you even better at taking care of others. If this caregiver matrix trap applies to you, then your challenge is to get yourself on as predictable a schedule as you can, with diet, exercise, and sleep-wake times.

Adjusting Your Mindset

If you're an older but also still relatively a novice trainee, then you need to realize that you are not going to develop a physique as fast as a younger person can, not even in comparison to someone in their 30s or 40s. Furthermore, if you are a retired competitor, you aren't going to progress as fast as you used to. So you can't train like you used to, or consume all those surplus calories as though you need them. This is one reason why some people in the masters' age group - who are actually in pretty good shape – end up looking like they're not in good shape. For instance, there are many regular training guys my age at my gym with middle-age paunches that they would rather not have.

We will discuss "diet" elements separately, but in terms of lifestyle considerations this is important to note here.

Exercise Trumps Diet

Many people in their 50s look to diets alone to control their weight: That is a mistake, and it is another reason I call this project *Physique After 50,* and not something like 'Diet After 50' or 'Weight-Loss After 50.' Exercise after age 50 is *the key element* to weight-control and to keeping the effects of sarcopenia at bay.

John Foreyt, PhD, professor of medicine and psychiatry at Baylor College of Medicine in Houston, and director of its Nutrition Research Clinic, showed that exercise is more important than dieting for *sustainable* weight-loss. In one study, researchers followed people who wanted to lose weight. The subjects were in 3 different groups:

- Group 1 exercised and dieted
- Group 2 dieted without exercise
- Group 3 exercised without dieting.

After two years, *only the group that exercised without seriously dieting* was the one that maintained its weight-loss.

It's often true that, psychologically speaking, when people work out regularly they don't want to "blow it" by eating crappy food. Exercise likely provides added incentive to stick to a healthy eating regimen, and it helps establish regimented lifestyle routines in the first place. This tends to carry over into regimented mealtimes.

The Importance of Sleep for Quality of Life and Weight Control

Chronic sleep deprivation is not part of a lifestyle that supports health and fitness. The research on sleep consistently concludes that if you do not get enough quality and quantity of sleep, it makes you hungry, impotent, disinterested, hypertensive, and fat – just to name a few consequences. Adequate quality and quantity of sleep are crucial to recovery from exercise, and for overall daily and weekly rejuvenation.

There are also stark gender disparities in people with sleep issues as well. Women tend to suffer insomnia far more frequently and dramatically than men.

Sleep is vital to optimizing all the hormonal functions we need for the cosmetic effects we are pursuing when seeking a cosmetically improved physique after 50. The problem here is that disrupted sleep is also more common as we age. Therefore, we must pay even greater attention to sleep hygiene. People of all ages underestimate the value of effective sleep.

If you are serious about developing and maintaining a cosmetically pleasing physique after age 50, then you need to take quality of sleep seriously.

Sleep Hygiene

People ask me all the time *"What exactly is good sleep hygiene?"*

- **Good sleep-hygiene includes the little things like sleeping in a dark and cool room and avoiding bringing "work and worry" into bed with you**. "How" you do that is an individual variant you will need to develop, and then practice till it becomes habit. It's about establishing a bedtime ritual.

- Try to exercise earlier in the day, and not within three to four hours of bedtime. Find ways to wind down in those few hours before bedtime.

- Research is showing that it is not only better, but also practically crucial to keep the same sleep schedule seven days per week if possible.

- Inconsistency with sleep contributes to food and eating issues. The first things I address in individuals with binge-eating disorders are their sleep habits and sleep hygiene. Almost all of them are lacking in this area. They sleep in on weekends. They can't fall asleep at night. They like to party or stay up late when they can. I instruct them to aim for regular sleep and wake times. Most of them resist. I also instruct them to stop sleeping in late and get up at the same time every single day, – no matter what time they got to bed the night before. Stay up for an hour or two *and then*, if you want to go back to bed, do so. And yet almost every single one of them would not follow this simple direction consistently enough to create healthy change.

- We know melatonin (commonly known as the sleep hormone) is suppressed by light, especially sky-blue sunlight. Exposure to artificial light at night disrupts melatonin production and delays the onset of sleep. Just two hours of iPad or tablet use at maximum brightness is enough to suppress normal nighttime release of melatonin. Two hours of computer use closer to your sleep time not only lowers melatonin secretion but also enhances cognitive attention, lighting up the brain to "be awake." In reality, you shouldn't be looking at any "glowing screens" at least one to two hours before retiring to bed to sleep. Television viewing may be fine, but backlit screens like tablets and cell phones should be avoided. If you are going to read close to bedtime, then hard copy books or magazines are the better choice.

- **You can't wind down and seek stimulus at the same time.** Social media surfing just before bedtime is a lot like trying to sleep while listening to heavy metal music playing at maximum volume. Avoid the enticement of social media, and other mental and emotional stimulus close to bedtime. This is not the time to be answering emails or sending tweets.

- Your natural rhythm will present a particular window of opportunity for falling asleep. If you miss that window because you are doing something with a close-up glowing screen, or "staying up past your bedtime," then you may end up tossing and turning most of the night. You need to establish a winding down ritual in order to invite that natural opportunity for sleep to come. **Winding down is distinctly better than tuning in.**

- You need to also keep in mind that your immune system uses sleep time to do its housecleaning and repair work! If you want to remain healthy and free from colds, flu bugs and everything else, you need good quality of sleep.

Other No-Brainer Basics

Let's tie some general points together now to create an overall checklist for your reference. To be able to accomplish and sustain a better physique after 50 means approaching things a little differently than you likely have been doing. It *also* definitely means approaching things differently than you might have when you were younger. **The better you are treating yourself from the inside-out, you greatly improve how good you can look from the outside-in.** You must develop healthy habits that nurture healthy well-being of mind, body, and spirit. Here are a few no-brainer basics that you should establish if you seek a better physique after

50.

- Eat breakfast every single day, preferably at the same time every single day.

- Avoid snacking between scheduled meal-times or scheduled snacks – stick to regimens and routines for your eating.

- Work toward a sustainable weight where you feel good and function optimally. Don't make it about arbitrary numbers on a scale.

- Work out regularly, whether you feel like it or not.

- Sleep seven to eight hours per night. If you have interrupted sleep, just stay in bed and put yourself into "relax mode." Keep regular sleep and wake times as much as you can.

- Don't smoke. If you smoke, make priority efforts to quit.

- Drink in moderation. Similar to the above point – there's nothing wrong with enjoying a drink here and there. But try to keep it to once per week, holidays and vacations. You serve your body well by imbibing in alcohol as a treat, not as a daily lifestyle habit.

- Sugar also in moderation. Try to limit

desserts, sugared soft drinks and other sugary ingestibles to once per week. Sugar is especially hard on bodies after age 50.

- Don't hoard your emotions. By age 50 you should be able to feel and process your emotions. It is unhealthy for your body AND your overall well-being if you can't. Medicating emotions is not a healthy alternative.

- Aim to finish your workout feeling energized and/or invigorated – never exhausted and spent.

- Your exercise regimen should serve to help relieve your stress, not add to it.

- Undertraining is better than overtraining.

- Consistency is more important than intensity.

The Modified Capital "S" Directive

I first came across a variation of the Capital-S Directive in one of Michael Pollan's books. His directive is not the same as mine, but it's very similar. Reinhard Engals wrote a whole book on a very similar theme, called *The No S Diet.*

I have discussed the Capital "S" directive in a few of my projects. It's a general guideline for eating habits and lifestyle habits, that reflect further on the "No Brainer Basics" section above.

Adapt the Abel Capital "S" directive and stick to it. This directive is very simple:

- No Snacks

- No Second Helpings

- No Spirits (alcohol)

- No Sweets

- No Sugars (artificial sweeteners are just fine)

- No Supersizing

- No Splurges, except for one day of the week that starts with "S," or is a "Special" occasion. (This day is also when you could enjoy some alcohol.)

- Add to this "S" directive - Sleep is a priority and...

- No Smoking!

This Capital "S" directive is a great accompaniment to any diet strategy you may be following. It is a fantastic directive to put in place to make any diet strategy effective.

The Body Thrives on Routine

Keep this Abel-ism in mind as well: "The Body Thrives on Routine." Regular sleep times, wake times, meal times, and training times – these all become even more important as you age (for hormonal balance and optimum biochemistry.) The more regimented you are with these things, the more your body "appreciates it" and responds accordingly.

Chapter 7.

How to Balance Rest and Recovery

The Base Hit Strategy

Baseball is a game of strategy. Home runs are fun to watch, but teams know they can't win a pennant surviving on a steady diet of them. The idea is to move runners around the bases, and the most reliable way to consistently do that is with base hits. You don't need home runs to win. In fact, in the last five years, two of the teams that reached the World Series actually hit the *fewest* home runs during the season (The 2012 Giants and the 2014 Royals.)

I was once at a baseball game sitting near someone who didn't understand the game's strategy very well. A batter laid down a bunt to advance a runner. The batter was thrown out at first base but the runner advanced from second base to third base. I remember the lady saying to her friends, "Why are they congratulating him? He got out at first base?"

You can successfully apply this same approach to your regular exercise regimen, especially after age 50

There's no reason to kill yourself in the gym. Research is mounting that clearly shows that less intense exercise, and less time-consuming exercise, have health benefits almost as great as the most demanding training protocols. In other words, training longer and harder adds only minimal benefit. Furthermore, it is now being shown that excessive exercise takes a health toll on the body beyond a risk of injury. And as we know from CrossFit®, ridiculously high intensity training risks kidney-related issues like rhabdomyolysis. It's simply not necessary to exercise till you drop, or exercise till exhaustion, although it makes for popular TV programming like Biggest Loser.

Constant maximal efforts in your workouts after age 50 can exhaust you and burn you out if you aren't careful.

Applying intensity to your workout regimen is all about nuance and subtlety. Every kind of stress in your life—physical, mental, and emotional—taps into your overall energy reserve. It's simply not realistic, or wise for that matter, to think you can give a "home run" max effort in every single workout.

The more stress you have in your life outside of your exercise regimen, and the busier your days, the more you should be applying the base hit strategy to your exercise regimen.

The truth is that it's not just how hard you work out that matters; it's how hard and efficiently you work out. This means understanding biofeedback and application of intensity. You can look at it like this: Applied intensity is a lot like using the gas pedal in your car. It's not always meant to be "pedal to the metal" to get to your destination. Embrace the benefits of the "base hit-strategy" and keep your "home-run-ego" in check.

The base hit strategy may mean training at a slower pace, or with lighter loads than usual, or doing fewer sets than usual, or all three of those. It may also mean applying this strategy for one workout day, or for a whole week of workouts.

It's okay to back off training intensity today so that you can train again tomorrow.

This may not sound "hardcore." But "hardcore" seldom applies to real people with real lives, who need to be flexible and vary the intensity of their training regimens. I will often assign people a base hit week with dialed back workout intensity, only to have them write me a week later saying they can't believe the difference.

The late strength expert Charlie Francis was onto something: He said, **"It is always better to undertrain than to overtrain**. *You will still produce adaptive stress, but maybe not to the same degree."*

Once you overtrain, your body's resilience plummets and fights to retain a balance. The rush to get more done "right now" because of excitement and enthusiasm leads to consequences down the road; often burnout. On the other hand, smaller central nervous system demands, spread over a longer period of time, result in more acceptance and greater improvement.

It's ok to back off training pace when you just aren't "feeling it" in the gym on a given day. What you need to remember and embrace is that training *consistency* is more important than *intensity*, especially after 50. For our age group, constantly going all-out leads to eventual burnout.

A base hit mindset strategy keeps you training consistently, and relieves the pressure of feeling you have to over-achieve in the gym every workout. You no longer have the pressure of thinking it's a home run intensity effort or else a wasted effort. That is no way to look an exercise lifestyle.

Trainees, who work very hard and consistently, increase their performance when they're allowed a bit of extra rest and recuperation. "More work," or "harder work," is seldom the answer to stalled progress for someone who trains hard and consistently already. This is especially true of an advanced trainee with many years of training under their belt. Active recovery, in the form of the "base hit mindset strategy," fits this application as well – whether that application is for a single workout, or a whole training week. In baseball, a base hit keeps the inning alive, and keeps the offense on the field. A base hit workout, with its dialed back pace and load, keeps you and your program in concert.

Avoiding Extended Time Off

When should you take a day off, or what should you do on off days from weight workouts? What about extended time off?

Regular exercise is important after age 50. If you are on an actual training program, then off-days will be laid out for you. This project, for instance, comes with my own 6-Day version of PA50 program, as well as a beginner program that is only two to three days per week. In the beginner version I will often add other forms of exercise so the trainee can get used to the regular discipline of consistent training.

Extended times off—as in two to three weeks—are less effective, and not recommended after age 50. The reasons here are (a) you aren't training as hard anyway (and shouldn't be), so extended layoffs for recovery shouldn't be necessary; and (b) it is much *much* harder to get back into shape after a layoff once you are over 50.

As an example, I formerly never worked out on vacations. That was always time off of from diet and training for me, since I did those things for a living. But after I turned 50, I found I now have to make time to workout on vacations or my joints hurt more, and I am much stiffer every day. It takes much longer to get back to where I was before a break. So now I pretty much work out even on vacations, even if it's a reduced regimen.

Strike a balance between establishing a routine and being overzealous with your training efforts, since you can more easily overdo things after age 50 than in previous years. After age 50, it doesn't take much to throw you off balance, tapping too far into your energy reserve.

Very often, you will need to back off your training pace for a workout or two, or the loads you use, or the intensity you apply to your workout. If you have been overdoing your workouts for any reason, then you shouldn't be worried about taking a day, a week, or sometimes even two to three weeks off from training if you think you need it.

Days-off from training should be built into your training program. If you are on a good solid training program that fits where you are at conditioning-wise; then there should be no reason to 'need' extended time off from training. Of course there are exceptions, and this is where having a reliable Coach's advice becomes invaluable.

If you think you need to take a long break off from training, then clearly you have been doing something wrong, so you should seek guidance from a Coach. At our age, if your training has burned you out, you will likely know it. It won't hurt you to take time off if you are burned out, while not taking time off certainly could hurt you! Sometimes you need a break. Sometimes you just need to "reboot" the system. So, mentally and emotionally speaking, sometimes getting away from something you love to do is a good way of reminding you how much you love it.

Chapter 8.

Bodypart-Specific Training Tweaks

Every so often, my comments about training elicit that confused "puppy dog look" from people. Today at the gym, someone was commenting on my physique and relating it to some barbell exercise he and his partner were doing. When I commented that I don't do barbell exercises anymore, and that I only use dumbbells, machines and cables, they were confused and gave me that "how is that possible?" look.

Everyone my age with a history of training with weights, or a background in any sport where they competed seriously or on a high level, are all going to have "war stories" to share. I know people at my age getting hip, knee, or even shoulder replacements. Shoulder replacement surgery pretty much ends any ability to continue serious weight training. Back, hip, knee, neck and shoulder problems—and just overall stiffness—are all quite common in our age group. These realities mean paying even closer attention to exercises that help, versus exercises that hurt. And it *should* also necessitate greater attention to proper program design and implementation for our age group. Just showing up at the gym is usually not enough; and it's especially not enough if developing or enhancing your physique after 50 is your goal.

If you are a retired competitor, you need to resist the temptation to try to do things you think you "ought" to be able to do, based on how you did them when you were younger. Be realistic about this and things will go better. I've witnessed several former competitors get one injury after another as they age, because they keep comparing their new reality with "what they used to be able to do." That can be a recipe for injury and frustration. I often refer to Sylvester Stallone tearing his pec by training his experience instead of training his age. It can be a hard lesson to learn, but many of you with a high performance background need to learn and heed this lesson, before you have to learn it the hard way.

No one can use the same workout training volume they could when they were younger; and this specifically applies to a bodybuilder's workout volume. Trying to do 20 sets for one body part in one workout places far too much joint stress on any over-50 body part. It is simply just too much volume and too much tissue breakdown to be able to recover from. However, I have found for the advanced over-50 trainee like myself, it is still possible for higher volume body part workload, if that volume is spread out over the course of the whole week. Remember that training for sculpting a physique after 50 begins and ends with joint protection.

How to Tweak your Training (General)

Tweak is another word for substituting one exercise for another similar one, used to keep your program "alive." A prime example would be substituting Bulgarian Split Squats for Single-leg Leg Press, if, say for instance, a leg press machine isn't available at the time. Tweaking is something done within the overall context of a program.

Below I am going to offer you my take on the best options of exercises to use for each body part, and even some to avoid or minimize. You can refer to this list for appropriate "tweaks." The list below is certainly not meant to be exhaustive. Think of it more as a beneficial starting guideline to body part exercise choices for the Physique After 50 crowd.

The 'avoid or minimize list' is all about erring on the side of caution, considering the Physique After 50 demographic and its most common injuries and chronic conditions. The "Avoid or minimize" lists are all about "prevention."

Let's add some common sense here. If it hurts, don't do it. I'm not talking about the kind of discomfort from a muscle exerting force. I'm talking about pain. Anyone should be able to tell the difference. Typically, true pain is felt in the joints not the muscles.

Legs: Best Options

Squat machines | Leg press machines | DB Squats with DBs hanging at your sides | DB lunges or split squat variations, with DBs hanging at your sides | Leg extension and leg curl machines | DB deadlift, with DBs hanging at your sides

Avoid or minimize:

Barbell squat | Barbell deadlift, especially Sumo version | Adductor/abductor machine (they simply don't offer much in terms of adaptive stress) | Explosive stuff, like jumping with weights

Back: Best Options

Any pulldown variations | Any seated row or cable row machine variations | Any supported row variations | DB Bent rows, with DBs (toward the side of the foot; not directly in front at the bottom of the movement) | Any one arm row variations | One arm pulldown variations

Avoid or Minimize:

Romanian deadlifts (RDL) | Barbell bent rows | T-Bar rows

Chest: Best Options

Any DB Press or DB fly variations | Any chest press machine or fly machine variations | Cable crossover or other cable chest exercises | Pec deck | Push-ups

Avoid or Minimize:

Barbell bench press | Barbell incline press (especially if you have any history of shoulder or elbow issues | Any explosive push up variations

Shoulders: Best Options

Any Seated DB shoulder Press variation | Any shoulder press *machine* variation | Any DB or cable front raise variation | Any DB or cable or machine lateral raises variation | Any DB or cable bent lateral variation | DB or cable upright rows | Any shrug variation, other than barbell | Any rear delt machine variation, including cables or tubing | Push ups (they are a combination shoulder/chest movement)

Avoid or Minimize:

Any Barbell shoulder press | Barbell upright rows | Barbell shrugs | Battling ropes

Triceps: Best Options

Any one- or two-arm cable triceps pushdown variation | Any seated triceps machine | Lying or seated two-arm DB extensions | Overhead rope extensions | One arm DB cross chest extension | One arm DB overhead extension | Cable triceps kickbacks | Triceps dips between benches (with caution. See below.)

Avoid or Minimize:

Parallel bar dips (hard on elbows and shoulder joint), but ok if you have no issues in these areas. Use good judgement for any dip variation.

Biceps: Best Options

Single or double arm versions of:

Seated DB alternate curls | Any cable or curls machine variations | DB Hammer Curls | DB Zottman Curls |

Preacher curl variation | Any concentration curls variation

Avoid or Minimize:

Barbell Cheat Curls (These present a lumbar spine risk, and compromise good shoulder position. If you love them and can do them pain-free, go ahead.

Chapter 9.

A Program for Physique After 50

In the appendix, I have program section where I give you three different training variations suitable for a trainee after age 50.

- A 2-3 day per week beginner program.
- A 3-6 day per week program (Hardgainer Solution*)
- A 6-Day program *based* on Hardgainer Solution

In my book, The Hardgainer Solution, I write about how anyone over 50 is automatically a hardgainer because of the realities of physiological, biochemical, and hormonal changes that take place at that age.

I have a beginner program in there, which is a straight sets program. "Straight sets" just means there are no biplexes or triplexes, in which two or three exercises are combined to become one set. In a straight sets program, you do *all* the sets of one exercise and then move on to the next exercise.

The beginner program is meant to be done only two to three days per week. It allows the over-50 trainee to get accustomed to doing resistance training, or reacquaint their body to it after a long layoff. Other days of the week for the beginner can be filled with other forms of exercise until the trainee can do more days of training, or progress to a higher level like the HGS program.

I have included an intermediate/advance program of 10 workouts taken directly from my *Hardgainer Solution*.

I have also included my own current personal *6-Day Physique After 50 Program*, also built on of the HGS Program.

All of these programs are based on training the whole body each workout. Whole body training has several general advantages that are outlined in the HGS book. For the over-50 trainee especially, however, whole body workouts have a systemic effect that will likely prevent overtraining and promote an overall positive metabolic effect.

Often, people over 50 are anxious about

beginning a weight training program because they fear having a heart attack. But really it's the people who don't exercise or take care of themselves nutritionally who are more likely to have heart attacks. As I outlined at the beginning of this project, research abounds about the benefits of resistance training as we age. Fearing health issues because of exercising doesn't make much sense unless your doctor has specifically outlined a reason why you should avoid exercise.

Conclusion

Rippetoe writes, "There is just something wrong with getting up every day and moving through your existence with the least possible effort."

And now at my age, I also see in other people the consequences of living the path of least resistance. I'd rather live well, than live long, if those extended years mean being unhealthy, out of shape, and with a low quality of life.

My glory days are right now.

Developing healthy habits is imperative. Look around you at the people who don't do these things before age 50, and see how limited they are by the time they reach their 50s. Life is busier and more stressful now than ever, but doesn't have to be. Being busy and stressed is all the more reason to make time to work out and eat right. Busy and stressed with no release leads to ill-health and use of coping mechanisms such as drinking, or taking prescription drugs for mood or sleep.

Remember the two guys I mentioned at the beginning of this book, who both look and feel great? These two gentlemen didn't even begin working out until their late 40s! They will admit that they don't know a lot when it comes to training. But they look fantastic. They are living proof that a little knowledge and a lot of discipline, underpinned with committed consistency, is the secret (if there is such a thing in training) to accomplishing and sustaining a physique after 50. They've adopted "body part" traditional bodybuilding training, and are involved in other physical activities. Their friends and acquaintances their age frequently ask them how they look so good. They answer that they weight train and they eat well. Yet the acquaintances who question them still seek simple answers through "magic" supplements, diets, or pills.

I poke fun at my own physique and my looks as the years pile up. I often say, "The older I get, the younger I used to be." But I can poke fun at myself because at my current age, I've never been happier. Your outer presentation says a lot about your inner health and well-being. Appreciate and respect the changes that come with age. Thinking you can fight these changes, or being sad and depressed over them, doesn't make any sense for health and well-being.

Muscle recovery, strength and flexibility do not get better and improve with age, yet attitude and proper disposition can. Focus on the positive. Emphasize what you're able to do. **Aim to get as much as you can out of what you can do, devote yourself sincerely to it, and you'll be amazed how far you can take it, if you're consistent.**

If you're an older person and just starting a training program, your ability to make progress is affected by several factors that younger trainees take for granted – like sleep, nutrition, recovery, and stress. Set different expectations if you are an older trainee seeking cosmetic physique changes.

You don't have to just be a passive recipient of the aging process.

We over-50 trainees have a diminished response to the stress of physical exertion due to the real but sobering fact that we have far lower levels of the anabolic hormones that aid recovery and adaptation. This, as much as your list of chronic conditions and injuries, has the potential to limit your progress. Proper program design becomes even more important for these reasons. Keep this reality in mind as you work toward accomplishing a better-sculpted physique after 50. The "no pain no gain" motto does not apply to the over-50 age group.

The body is like any other fine machine. It requires regular and routine maintenance and protection so that the years don't wear it out.

Let me conclude by repeating: Longevity is more than how long you live, but how well you live. Most of us have been socialized into expecting far too little of the aging body and physique, and are being convinced to just sit back and let aging happen. Worse, resisting aging only brings anguish, because it's futile to fight certain realities. But by choosing to improve yourself, you stay youthful. To expect more than passive acceptance from your aging physique marks the difference between having "golden years" versus choosing to experience a "Platinum Club" quality existence.

Physique after 50 (PA50) – working out and exercising to sculpt and enhance your physique— can be challenging, but that makes it all the more fun and intriguing. It has for me. Attitude determines altitude. Let's start a movement – a movement away from passive acceptance of Golden Years. Let's set an example of active and invigorated membership in the Platinum Club, where all are welcome, and age is not a setback; it's a gift.

Appendix

3-Day Per Week Beginner Program

Rules of Application

- This is a whole body training program.

- Although there are four workouts, this is a 3-Day program.

- The days of the week you train do not matter, but avoid training two days in a row.

- Do not train to failure.

- Properly warm up before beginning your workout. This includes a general preparation phase as well as actual physical rehearsal (light warm up sets, etc.)

Conditioning Into the Program:

- Train two to three days per week. You can start at two workouts each week, then move up to three.

- You can also begin by only doing Workout 1 over and over, then Workout 1 and 2, then 1 through 3, and then finally cycling through all four.

KEY:

BW	Bodyweight
DB	Dumbbell
EA	Each Arm
EL	Each Leg

Workout 1

	Sets	Reps
Leg press	3	15-20
Lying leg curls	3	20, 15, 12
Hack squats or DB Squats	1	20
Seated rows	2	15, 12
Bent rows	1	12-15
Machine shoulder press	3	15, 12, 10
DB or BB upright rows	2	15, 10-12
Machine chest press	3	8-10
Flat flys	2	15, 10-12
DB concentration curls	1	15-20
Alternating hammer curls	1	10-12
Tricep pushdowns	2	10-12
One arm dumbbell extension	1	10-12

Workout 2

	Sets	Reps
BW or DB squats	3	25, 20, 15
Leg extensions	2	15-20
One arm rows	3	8-10
Pulldowns to chest	2	12-15
Incline DB press	2	15, 12
Pec dec or chest fly machine	1	15-20
Seated side laterals	3	15, 12, 10
Alternate DB press (shoulder)	1	12-15
Overhead rope extensions	1	12-15
One arm preacher curls	1	8-10
Sit ups of any kind	1	12-15

Workout 3

	Sets	Reps
Leg presses or hack squats	3	20, 15, 10-12
Lunges, alternating or single leg	2	10-12 EL
DB stiff legged deadlift	1	12-15
Flat DB press	3	8-12
Incline machine or DB press	1	12-15
Seated cable rows	3	15, 12, 10
Reverse grip pulldowns	1	10-12
Bent DB laterals or rear delt machine	2	12-15
Front DB alternate raises	1	12-15 EA
Lying DB tricep extensions	2	12-15
Standing barbell or cable curls	2	10-15
Tricep pushdowns	1	10-15
Dumbbell concentration curls	1	10-12

Workout 4

	Sets	Reps
Leg extensions	3	20, 15, 10
Leg curls	3	15, 12, 10
One legged leg press	1	15-20 EL
Incline DB or incline machine press	2	8-12
Seated machine or cable flys	1	8-10
One arm DB rows	1	8-10
Close grip pulldowns	2	10-12
Machine shoulder press	3	15, 12, 10
Bent DB laterals	1	15-20
One arm DB extensions	1	10-15
Incline alternate DB curls	1	8-10
Standing barbell curls	1	10-12
One arm pushdowns	1	12-15

Hardgainer Solution Workouts

Rules of Application

You'll notice these are also whole body workouts. That gives you a lot of flexibility in terms of how many days per week you train.

You could work out three days a week, and just pick three workouts to go through again and again. Or you try a two-week split that looked like this:

Week 1						
Monday	Tuesday	Wednesday	Thursday	Friday	Saturday	Sunday
Workout 1		Workout 2		Workout 3		

Week 2						
Monday	Tuesday	Wednesday	Thursday	Friday	Saturday	Sunday
Workout 4		Workout 5		Workout 6		

Based on the above, on Week 3 you could start again at Workout 1, or you could simply continue to Workouts 7, 8, and 9, and not start repeating through the workouts until you'd gone through all ten of them. It's up to you.

That example assumes you're working out three days per week. Of course, you can also work out four days per week, five days per week, or six days per week, based on how you are feeling on the program.

I recommend that you condition into the program. This means don't jump straight into working out six days per week unless you have been doing that already. Instead, work your way up to this. In this way, these Hardgainer workouts can serve as a *bridge* between the 3-Day Physique After 50 Program and the 6-Day Physique After 50 Program.

Note also, that as part of conditioning into the program, you can stick with just one or two workouts at first, so that you can get used to the rhythm of performing complexes. That is not necessary, but it is an option.

Performing Complexes Correctly

As you look through the workouts you will notice that all of the exercises are grouped into either groups of two or three exercises like 'a' and 'b' (for two exercises), or 'a', 'b' and 'c' (for three). There are only a few exceptions where there is a single exercise not performed in a complex/superset of some sort.

These two or three individual exercises are grouped together by number. These groups are known as "complexes" and the idea is that exercise a), exercise b) and exercise c) of that complex are performed back to back. Performing two (or all three) of those exercises constitutes one set of a complex.

After a set, you rest until you are ready to repeat the set again, and ready to perform the two or three exercises again back to back. You repeat the total amount of sets prescribed before moving on to the next group of exercises (i.e. the next complex) and you execute the next complex in the same fashion.

I will illustrate with an example from "Workout 1" below:

Workout 1	Sets X Reps
1a) DB or BB Squats	5 X 5
1b) DB Incline Press	5 X 8-10
1c) DB or BB Upright Rows	5 X 20
2a) Pulldowns Behind the Head	4 X 12-15
2b) Two-Arm DB Curl	4 X 20
3a) One-Arm DB triceps extension	4 X 5-6
3b) Any sit up or leg raise variation	4 X 20

Exercise 1a), 1b) and 1c) represent your first complex.

You perform them all back to back and at an even pace for the amount of reps prescribed for each of the three exercises. In other words, you perform 5 reps of dumbbell or barbell squats, then immediately you perform 8-10 reps of dumbbell incline press, then immediately you perform 20 reps of dumbbell or barbell upright rows, then you rest, and that's one set. You have 4 more sets of this complex, for a total of 5. Then you move on to complex 2.

Workout 1

	Sets X Reps
1a) DB or BB Squats	5 X 5
1b) DB Incline Press	5 X 8-10
1c) DB or BB Upright Rows	5 X 20
2a) Pulldowns Behind the Head	4 X 12-15
2b) Two-Arm DB Curls	4 X 20
3a) One-Arm DB triceps extension	4 X 5-6 EA
3b) Any sit up or leg raise variation	4 X 12-20

Workout 2

	Sets X Reps
1a) Seated cable rows	5 X 15-20
1b) Triceps Dips Between Benches	5 X 15-20
2a) Seated Cable Flys	4 X 8-12
2b) Leg Extensions	4 X 20
3a) Seated DB Shoulder press	4 X 8-12
3b) Alternate Hammer Curls	4 X 5 EA
3c) Any sit ups or leg raise variation	3-4 X 12-20

Workout 3

	Sets X Reps
1) Incline DB Press	5 X 5
2a) Seated Side Laterals	4 X 20
2b) Straight Arm Pulldowns	4 X 15-20
2c) One-Leg Leg Press*	4 X 20
3a) Seated Alternate DB Curls	4 X 5-6 EA
3b) Lying Triceps extensions	4 X 12-15
3c) Continue One Leg Press as directed above	

* On these types of workouts, only do ONE SIDE of a unilateral movement unless otherwise indicated. So for exercise 2c) you will do left side one leg press the first round of sequence 2 and you will do the right side on the second round of sequence 2. So, one leg leg press will spill into exercise 3 in order to complete all 4 sets on each side

Workout 4

	Sets X Reps
1a) DB Bent Lateral Raises	5 X 12-15
1b) Fly DB Flys	5 X 8-10
1c) BW Bulgarian Split Squat*	5 X 20 EL
2a) Reverse Grip Pulldowns	4 X 8-10
2b) Continue Split Squat as above	20 EL
3a) One-Arm DB concentration curls	4 X 8-10
3b) One-Arm Reverse Grip Triceps Pushdowns	4 X 15-20

* Again this is a single side movement, so do right or left leg on the first round, then the other leg on the next round and continue till you've done all 5 sets for each leg

Workout 5

	Sets X Reps
1a) Cable Crossovers	5 X 15-20
1b) One-Arm DB Rows	5 X 5 EA
1c) DB Single Leg Lunges*	5 X 8-10 EL
2a) Front Alternate DB Raises	4 X 12-15
2b) Over Rope Triceps Extensions	4 X 12-15
2c) Continue left over Single Leg Lunges till all 5 sets	
3a) One-Arm Zottman Curls	4 X 5 EA
3b) Any sit up or leg raise variation	4 X 12-15

* Single leg lunge is done only one side per round, so left leg on the first round of 1c and right leg on the second round. Therefore this exercise continues into the next sequence until all 5 sets are complete.

Workout 6

	Sets X Reps
1a) Flat DB or BB Press	5 X 5
1b) DB Squats	5 X 5
2a) Seated DB Shoulder Press	4 X 5
2b) Alternating Pulldowns (palms face each other)	4 X 8-10
2c) Any sit ups or leg raise variation	4 X 15-20
3a) Triceps Pushdowns	4 X 8-10
3b) Standing Simultaneous DB Curls	4 X 20

Workout 7

	Sets X Reps
1a) Cable or machine rear delts	5 X 15-20
1b) Low Incline DB Flys	5 X 10-12
1c) DB or BB alternating lunges	5 X 5 EL
2a) One-Arm DB Triceps Extension	4 X 15-20
2b) One-Arm Preacher Curls	4 X 15-20
3a) One-Arm Reverse Grip Pulldowns	4 X 8-10
3b) Any sit up or leg raise variation	4 X 12-15

Workout 8

	Sets X Reps
1a) Leg Press	5 X 20
1b) Two-Arm DB Front Raises	5 X 20
1c) Lying Triceps Extensions	5 X 5
2a) One-Arm Low Pulley Rows	4 X 12-15 ES
2b) Any sit ups or leg raise variation	4 X 12-15
2c) High Incline DB Press	4 X 20
3) Standing Single Arm DB Curls	4 X 15 EA

Workout 9

	Sets X Reps
1a) DB Concentration Curls	5 X 5
1b) Cable or Tubing One Arm Triceps Kickback	5 X 20
1c) One-Arm Cable Side Laterals	5 X 15 ES
2a) DB Sumo Squat	4 X 20
2b) High Angle Seated Rows	4 X 15-20
3a) Low Incline DB flys	4 X 5
3b) Any sit ups or leg raise variation	4 X 12-15

Workout 10

	Sets X Reps
1a) Seated Machine Chest Press	5 X 12-15
1b) DB Bent Rows	5 X 8-10
1c) Any sit ups or leg raise variation	5 X 15-20
2a) DB or BB Shrugs	4 X 5
2b) Low Pulley Triceps Rope Extensions	4 X 12-15
2c) Single Leg Reverse Lunges*	4 X 20 EL
3a) One-Arm DB Hammer Curls	4 X 5 EA

3b) Continue Single Leg Reverse Lunges till all 4 sets each side are completed

* Single side movements like these are done only one side per round, so right side on the first round, left side on the second round. This means this exercise will be continued into the next sequence till all four sets are complete.

6-Day Physique After 50 Program

APPLICATION & INSTRUCTION

- This program builds off of my *Hardgainer Solution* protocol, but is slightly different.

- **No one in the Physique Over 50 demographic should be training to failure on any exercise.** That should be a hard and fast rule, but even if treated as "relative" you <u>especially</u> don't want to train to failure on a whole body program that is six days per week! Always leave something in the tank, exercise to exercise. Feel "challenged" within the rep ranges you are working in, and that is the guideline.

- This program takes a whole body approach, but with one "load emphasis and focus" day for each bodypart, where on that day you will do two exercises instead of one for that specific bodypart. That first exercise is for 3-4 sets of 5 reps (that's the load emphasis) of a compound movement of some kind.

- After that first exercise on a load focus day, any exercise can be done for rep ranges that surf the curve at 6-8 reps, 10-12 reps, 12-15 reps, or 15-20 reps. Just mix it up and make sure at least one time per week each bodypart is hit with each rep range above.

- The day after this load day for a specific bodypart, that bodypart is rested completely the next day.

- Day 6 is a "sets of 5" approach that is lighter and easier, in order to support the other five days of the week. No leg training is done on Day 6. After age 50, hitting legs four days of the week is more than enough stimulation.

- The **structure** is as follows:

  - Day 1: Legs emphasis
  - Day 2: Back emphasis
  - Day 3: Chest emphasis
  - Day 4: Whole body emphasis
  - Day 5: Delts emphasis

150

- Day 6: Sets of 5, with load emphasis, but lighter and easier.

- Note that on Day 6 you do not train legs or shoulder movements. So Days 4 and 6 are quicker workouts. This is deliberate to factor in recovery needs when training six days per week for the trainee who is over 50 years of age.

- Here, then, is what a week might look like:

Day 1	Day 2	Day 3	Day 4	Day 5	Day 6	Day 7
Two **Legs** exercises	Rest Legs. Two **Back** Exercises.	Rest Back. Two **Chest** Exercises.	Rest Chest. Two **Whole Body** Exercises.	Two **Delts** Exercises.	Overall Load Emphasis with Sets of 5. Rest Legs & Delts	**Rest Day.**

- The strategy is outlined above, but the tactical application can vary from biplexes to triplexes. There need be no specific rules about that, or sequence to it, other than usually the first exercise of each bodypart focus day is done on its own, with only GPP warmups for the other half of the body between sets. For instance, after the first few sets on Leg emphasis day, you would do GPP warmups for the upper body. On Day 2 and Day 3, between sets of the first exercise you would do GPP warm up sets for lower body. You can see videos of the GPP protocol at

151

http://scottabelfitness.com/warmups (making sure to watch part two, linked in the notes.)

- The bodyparts within a biplex or triplex can be combined in any order. In fact it is a good idea to mix it up, workout to workout.

- For PA50 trainees, training implements should consist almost entirely of dumbbells, machines, and cables. If you like barbell work, and feel no joint pain from using barbells then go ahead, but in terms of preventative maintenance and longevity for training, dumbbells, cables, and machines make the most sense by far for the trainee over 50 years of age.

- Avoid jarring movements, plyos, and ballistic movements.

- Training Note: Often, over-50 trainees may find that two leg exercises on Day 1 is too many when combined with the rest of the week's training volume, and when training 6 days per week. I myself removed the second leg exercise from Day 1, once I began my post-workout power walks. Feel it out and adapt accordingly. Listen to your body.

- Also, for me personally, I do not do abs/core work, and where you see abs/core work below I actually do rotator cuff work. See this video for a demo of that: http://scottabelfitness.com/rotatorcuff

- As a personal preference of my own, on the day before a "load focus day" for a specific bodypart, I prefer to use lighter weights and higher reps for that bodypart. For instance, since Day 3 is a load day for chest, on Day 2 right before chest day, I prefer to use lighter weights and higher reps for all my chest work.

- I also now cycle my arm work, so that on one day I do four sets for either biceps or triceps, but the next day only do three sets. So if on one training day I do four sets for triceps I will only do three sets for biceps and vice versa. The exceptions are if I choose to begin Day 4 with arm work, and on Day 6 as well, since the next day after day 6 is a complete rest day.

- These notes are just examples of "tweakology" and how I have tweaked the program based on my own ongoing biofeedback.

In the program breakdown below, I have included the "skeleton" version of this program (where instead of specific exercises you just see options, such as "Any back exercise" or "Any chest exercise"), and after this version I have included an "example" version where every exercise is filled in.

PA50 Program Breakdown

Day 1:
Legs Emphasis

Begin with GPP for lower body, since legs is the primary emphasis and first exercise

Exercise 1

1a) Any Squat Variation   3-4 X's 5 reps

1b) Just GPP warm ups for upper body between sets, slow and steady

Exercise 2

2a) A second leg exercise   4 X's 10-12

2b) Any back exercise   4 X's 15-20

2c) Any chest exercise   4 X's 12-15

Exercise 3

3a) Any shoulder exercise   4 X's 10-12

3b) Any biceps exercise   4 X's 10-12

Exercise

4a) Any triceps exercise   4 X's 12-15

4b) Any abs/core exercise   4 X's 12-15

Day 2:
Back Emphasis
No Leg Work

Begin with GPP for upper body, since back is the first exercise and load focus

Exercise 1

1a) Any Back exercise   3-4 X's 5 reps

1b) Just general GPP for lower body between sets, slow and steady

Exercise 2

2a) A second back exercise   4 X's 10-12

2b) Any shoulder exercise   4 X's 12-15

2c) Any triceps exercise   4 X's 12-15

Exercise 3

3a) Any biceps exercise   4 X's 12-15

3b) Any chest exercise   4 X's 15-20

Exercise 4

4) Any abs/core work   4 X's 12-15

Day 3:
Chest Emphasis
No Back Work

Begin with GPP for upper body since chest is the first exercise and bodypart focus

Exercise 1
1a) Any chest exercise   3-4 X's 5
1b) GPP for lower body between sets

Exercise 2
2a) A second chest exercise   4 X's 8-10
2b) Any shoulder exercise   4 X's 12-15
2c) Any leg exercise   4 X's 12-15

Exercise 3
3a) Any biceps exercise   4 X's 12-15
3b) Any triceps exercise   4 X's 12-15

Exercise 4
4) Any abs/core exercise   4 X's 12-15

Day 4:
Whole Body Emphasis
No Chest Work

Begin with total body GPP first

Exercise 1

1a) Any Leg Exercise	5 X's 15, 12, 10, 8, 6*
1b) Any Shoulder Exercise	4 X's 10-15
1c) Any Triceps Exercise	4 X's 12-15

Exercise 2

2a) Any Biceps exercise	4 X's 10-12
2b) Any Back exercise	4 X's 10-12

Exercise 3

3a) Any abs/core exercise	4 X's 12-15

* Note: On this day I may vary the leg work repetition schemes and maybe do all 5 sets at 20 reps, or 15 reps, or 12 reps, etc. It really depends what biofeedback my legs give me in the first set or two. If the legs feel tired I don't progress the load very much.

Day 5:
Delts + Whole Body Emphasis

Begin with GPP for upper body, since delts are the first exercise and the bodypart focus.

Exercise 1

1a) Any Delt Press   3-4 X's 5 reps

1b) GPP for lower body between sets

Exercise 2

2a) Any other delts exercise   4 X's 6-8, or 8-10

2b) Any chest exercise   4 X's 12-15

Exercise 3

3a) Any leg exercise   4 X's 8-10

3b) Any triceps exercise   4 X's 10-12

3c) Any back exercise   4 X's 12-15

Exercise 4

4a) Any biceps exercise   4 X's 15-20

4b) Any abs/core exercise   4 X's 15-20

Day 6:
Load Day Upper Body
No Delts or Leg Work

Begin with GPP for Upper Body.

Exercise 1
1a) Any Chest Press Variation   3 X's 5 reps
1b) GPP for lower body between sets

Exercise 2
2a) Any Back exercise   3 X's 5 reps
2b) Any Triceps Variation   3 X's 6-8

Exercise 3
3a) Any Biceps Curls   3 X's 5 reps
3b) Any abs/core exercise   3 X's 12-15

* Additional Notes for Day Six

This day can vary in terms of application **as long as the emphasis stays on heavier loads for 3 working sets of 5 reps.** (See my own sample workout below. For Day 6 I included to examples.)

I often combine the chest with back and then do the GPP for lower body between sets, turning the first complex into a triplex. Or, I will put the biceps curls with the chest exercise first, or other variations.

In total this often breaks down to 5 sets of 5 reps in total for these exercises, as there are usually at least 2 warm up sets for each exercise on Day 6.

This is more or less "a feeder day" for the following week. So the sets of 5 reps are still load focused, but a touch lighter than the actual weights used on the load focus day for these bodyparts.

I mix this day up a lot but always start with the chest press variation.

A Sample Week
of My Actual Workouts

(…to illustrate the application of this PA50 6-Day Program)

Sample Day 1:

Legs + Whole Body Emphasis *

Begin with GPP for lower body, since legs is the primary emphasis and first exercise.

Exercise 1

1a) Squat Machine at gym   4 X's 5 reps
1b) GPP for upper body between sets

Exercise 2

2a) Low Row Machine   4 X's 15-20
2b) Machine Preacher Curls   4 X's 15-20
2c) Machine Incline Chest Press   4 X's 12-15

Exercise 3

3a) Seated DB Shoulder Press   4 X's 15
3b) Reverse One-Arm Triceps Pushdowns   3 X's 15

Exercise 4

4a) Rotator Cuff Work (Internal Rotations)   4 X's 5-6 EA
4b) Anterior Reaches Variations   4 X's 5-8 EL

Note for this day:

As outlined in the application instructions, I myself only do one leg exercise on this day, simply because this time of year I go for power walks daily and the area around my home has a lot of hills.

In the winter, this workout will go back to two leg exercises for me.

This is an example of reading and gauging biofeedback and acting in accordance with it. This day still stays true to "load emphasis" for the leg work.

Sample Day 2:
Back Emphasis
No Leg Work

Begin with GPP for upper body since back is the first exercise and bodypart focus.

Exercise 1
1a) Seated Cable Rows　　　　　　　　4 X's 5 reps
1b) Cable Crossovers　　　　　　　　　4 X's 15-20
1c) Two-Arm DB Front Shoulder Raises　4 X's 20,15,12,10

Exercise 2
2a) One-Arm DB Rows　　　　　　　　4 X's 6
2b) One-Arm Cable Kickbacks　　　　4 X's 12

Exercise 3
3a) 1-Arm DB Concentration Curls　　3 X's 8
3b) GPP for lower body between sets

Exercise 4
4) Rotator Cuff Work (External Rotations)　4 X's 12 EA

Note for this day:

Usually I just isolate the first exercise for sets of 5, but today I mixed it up and created a triplex of heavy seated rows with two lighter chest and shoulder exercises.

This is just following the Abel Principle of "keeping it alive"!

After being on this program for about two years now, this is another example of personal "tweakology." I want to include what I am "actually doing" as an example within masterclass program design, and how it can be varied in application and while still ultimately sticking to the methodology and overall program design.

I wouldn't do this every week, but it is what I did *this* week.

Sample Day 3:
Chest Emphasis
No Back Work

Begin with GPP for upper body since chest is the first exercise and bodypart focus.

Exercise 1
1a) Low Incline DB Press   4 X's 5 reps
1b) GPP for Lower Body between sets

Exercise 2
2a) Hammer Machine Chest   4 X's 8-10
2b) DB Alternating Lunges   4 X's 8-10 EL
2c) DB Shrugs   4 X's 10-15

Exercise 3
3a) Alternating Hammer Curls   4 X's 12-15
3b) Triceps Pushdowns   3 X's 15

Exercise 4
4) Rotator Cuff Work (internal rotations) 4 X's 8-10 EA

Sample Day 4:

Whole Body Emphasis
No Chest Work

Begin with whole body GPP since lower and upper body will be mixed.

Exercise 1

1a) Horizontal Leg Press   5 X's, 15,12, 10,10,10
1b) Rear Delt Machine   4 X's 12-15
1c) Triceps Machine Extensions   4 X's 8-10

Exercise 2

2a) Pulldowns to Chest   4 X's 12-15
2b) 2-Arm Cable Biceps Curls   3 X's 15

Exercise 3

3a) Rotator Cuff Work (external rotations) 4 X's 8-10 EA
3b) Anterior Reach Variations   4 X's 8 EL

Sample Day 5:
Delts + Whole Body Emphasis

Begin with GPP for Upper body since delts is the first exercise and bodypart focus.

Exercise 1

1a) Seated DB Shoulder Press   4 X's 5 reps

1b) GPP for lower body between sets

Exercise 2

2a) Seated Side Laterals   4 X's 8-10

2b) DB Squats   4 X's 10-12

Exercise 3

3a) Seated Chest Flys   4 X's 12-15

3b) BB Bent Rows   4 X's 12

3c) Triceps Low to High   3 X's 12-15
   Machine Cable Extensions

Exercise 4

4a) Single Arm Cable   3 X's 15
   Concentration Curls

4b) Rotator Cuff Work (internal rotations)   4 X's 5

Notes for this training day:

Since the following day, Day 6, is heavy load day including arm exercises, I only do 3 sets for both triceps and biceps on Day 5.

Sample Day 6 (Sample 1)
Load Emphasis
Sets of 5 for Chest/Back/Arms
No Shoulder Work, No Leg Work

Begin with GPP for upper body since upper body work is the only focus on this day.

Exercise 1

1a) Flat DB Bench Press   3 X's 5
1b) Alternating Cable Pull Ins   3 X's 5
1c) GPP for Lower Body as active rest between sets

Exercise 2

2a) Seated Alternate DB Curls   3 X's 5 EA
2b) Lying 2 Arm DB extensions   3 X's 6-8

Exercise 3

3a) Rotator Cuff Work (external rotations) 3 X's 10-12
3b) Anterior Reach Variations   3 X's 8 EL

Sample Day 6 (Sample 2)

One of my favorites!

Exercise 1

1a) Low Incline DB Press   3 X's 5
1b) GPP for lower body between sets

Exercise 2

2a) One-Arm DB Rows   3 X's 5*ES
2b) One-Arm DB Seated   3 X's 5*EA
     Triceps Extensions

Exercise 3

3a) Seated DB Alternate Curls   3 X's 5
3b) Rotator Cuff Work (external rotations) 3 X's 8

* Note: On this day for Exercise #2, I do one-arm DB rows
for left side, then go straight to the one-arm DB triceps
extensions for my left side; only then do I do the one-arm DB
Rows for my right arm, and then the one-arm DB triceps
extensions for my right arm. This creates a different kind of
bilateral innervation. Again, just a personal side note of
preference and "tweakology."

General Notes for Day 6:

Day 6 is considered a general support day for the other 5 days of the week. You don't do shoulders on Day 6, because delts were the focus on Day 5. And doing legs on Day 6 would likely be too much leg work, but it *is* "optional."

Even though Day 6 is a load-focus day, you go a bit 'lighter' in load than you would on the actual bodypart focus days for the rest of the week. You also train at a bit slower pace as well.

Remember, for Physique Over 50, recovery needs must be considered. And when you're training 6 Days per week with weights, that can push work capacity into overtraining if you train too heavy too often. So even though Day 6 is a load emphasis day, it's done lighter and easier in terms of intensity of application.

Thank you for taking the time to read this book.

To learn more, get announcements about new programs or new books, visit scottabelfitness.com.

DISCLAIMER AND/OR LEGAL NOTICES:

Every effort has been made to accurately represent this book and its potential. Results vary with every individual, and your results may or may not be different from those depicted. No promises, guarantees or warranties, whether stated or implied, have been made that you will produce any specific result from this book. Your efforts are individual and unique, and may vary from those shown. Your success depends on your efforts, background and motivation.

The material in this publication is provided for educational and informational purposes only and is not intended as medical advice. The information contained in this book should not be used to diagnose or treat any illness, metabolic disorder, disease or health problem. Always consult your physician or health care provider before beginning any nutrition or exercise program. Use of the programs, advice, and information contained in this book is at the sole choice and risk of the reader.